Kundalini & Kriya Yoga

by

Dharam Vir Mangla
M.Sc. M.Ed. PGDCA

Edited by
Raju Gupta

Published by:

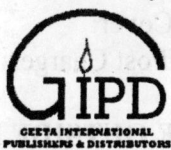

GIPD
GEETA INTERNATIONAL
PUBLISHERS & DISTRIBUTORS

GEETA INTERNATIOAL PUBLISHERS & DISTRIBUTORS
Phone # +91 +11-2242 9715
E-mail : dvmangla@hotmail.com
Web-site: www.geocities.com/godrealization

Copyright © 2003 and all rights reserved are with the author Dharam Vir Mangla & editor Raju Gupta. No part of this book may be reproduced in any form by any electronic or mechanical means, including information storage and retrieval systems, except for brief passages quoted in a book review.

Paper-Back	**ISBN # 81-901604-2-7**
Hard-Cover	**ISBN # 81-901604-3-5**

Publishers or Distributors interested in the publishing distribution of this book in different countries or in the translation right in different languages may contact the author by e-mail dvmangla@hotmail.com

Printed at: G.K. Fine Art Press, Delhi.
First Indian Edition: August 2003

PRICE IN INDIA
Paperback: Rs. 180.0
Hard Cover: Rs. 210.0
Book Post Charges: Rs. 20.0

PRICE OUTSIDE INDIA
Paperback: US $15.0
Hard Cover: US $18.0

Postage by Air + Handling Charges: US $3.0

PUBLISHED BY
GEETA INTERNATIONAL PUBLISHERS & DISTRIBUTORS IN INDIA
197 Geeta Apartments, Geeta Colony
Delhi-110031, INDIA
Phone # +91 +11 - 2242 9715
E-mail : dvmangla@hotmail.com

How to Order:
- Call +91 +11 - 2242 9715 or
- E-mail: dvmangla@hotmail.com or
- Browse URL: www.geocities.com/godrealization for direct and quick bank transfer of money.
- We execute the order on the same day after receiving payment by Bank Draft / Money Order / Telegraphic Transfer in the name of 'Geeta International Publishers & Distributors' or 'Dharam Vir Mangla'.

The contents given in this book are simply for the information to the readers. The practices of all the asanas, pranayama, exercises & mudras, meditations etc. should be done under the guidance of an experienced person. The author and the publishers are not responsible to any kind of loss or suffering to the readers. The court of jurisdiction will be only Delhi for any kind of dispute.

Dedicated to:

Sri Paramhansa Yogananda,
Sri Maharishi Patanjali
Sri Mahavatar Babaji
Sri Amar Jyoti Babaji
the Eternal Gurus

And

To all the Devoted Scientists
Doctors, Educationists, Yogis
and the Seekers of God & Truth

The suggestions and comments of the readers of this book are welcomed by the author through the e-mail:
dvmangla@hotmail.com

Also browse the
Website: http://www.geocities.com/godrealization

The author will try his best to respond the quarries of readers, if any.

If you feel this book is worth reading by others for the transformation of their soul, it will be your greatest divine service to God in this life to recommend this book to others or gift it to your friends, relatives and the seekers of God. There cannot be any other gift better then a soul-transforming book in their life, which can bring joy, bliss and happiness in their lives.

OTHER BOOKS BY THE SAME AUTHOR:

God & Self-Realization (Scientific & Spiritual View).

First Edition: October, 2002
Prices: Rs 180/- in India + Postage Rs. 20.0
                 US $ 15.00 Abroad + Postage US $ 3.0
Pages: 340
ISBN #:   81-901604-0-0

EXPECTED FUTURE BOOKS:
  1. How to Know God?
  2. Un-reality of The Universe
  3. Yoga for Perfect Health
  4. Illusion Delusion & Maya
  5. Miraculous Saints
  6. Dream & Death

CONTENTS

CHAPTERS	Page #
Contents	VIII-XIII
A Word	XV-XVI
About the Author	XVII
Preface	XVIII-XIX
How to Use this Book?	XX

1. Introduction to Yoga — 1-28
Prayer — 3
What is Yoga? — 4
The Power of the Mind — 5
The Ultimate Aim of Yoga — 7
The Types of Yoga — 10
Yog-Sutras of Maharishi Patanjali: — 12-18
   Yam, Niyama, Asana, Pranayam, Pratyahara
   Dharana, Dhyana and Samadhi.
Types of Samadhies: — 18
   Sabhikalpa & Nirvikalpa
Kundalini Shakti is the Spiritual Energy to — 20
   Unite Soul with God (Involution of soul)
Do Not be Afraid of Awakening of Kundalini — 22
Impact of Maya can be Removed after — 22
   Awakening of the Kundalini
Universe is a Great Thought in the Mind of God — 23
So Called Psychology is Not a Yogic Science — 25
Only Mental Renunciation and Not the Sanyias — 26
   is Needed by an Aspirant

2. The Basic Concepts of Kundalini Yoga — 29-60
Prayer — 31
The Theory of Kundalini Yoga — 32

What about Tibetan Buddhism?	38
Did Tibetans know about Kundalini?	38
Life Energy is Different from Physical Energies	39
Physical Body is not as it looks to our Senses	39
The Bodies of Men and other Living Beings are the Biggest Chemical Industries	40
Physical & Mental Works are Different	41
Do not Over-eat but must Do Regular Exercises	42
Many Prohibitions for an Aspirant	43
What are Granthis?	46
How to Increase the Reception and Retention of Life Force?	46
Vegetarian Food is Full of Life-Energy	49
Devotion & Love for God is Must for Awakening the Kundalini	50
Never Forget God	52
Om, Anahat Sounds & Laya Yoga	53
Harmony with Nature & Becoming One with All	55
Harmony with Five Gross Elements of Creation	56
Possession of a Human Soul by some other Soul	58

3. The Basics of Kriya & Bhakti Yoga   61-76

Prayer	62
Yogiraj Sri Mahavatar Babaji (Revivalist of the lost Science of Kriya Yoga)	63
The Basics of Kriya Yoga	66
The Basics of Bhakti Yoga	73

IX

4. The Life-Force, Nadis & Chakras   77-96

Prayer   78
Know Your Spinal Column   79
Body Cells Need Regular Recharging   80
What are *Nadis*?   80-83
    1. *Ida* 2. *Pingla* 3. *Sushumana*
Cross-section of Sushumana Nadi   82
The Symptoms of Sushumana Nadi Activation   83
Our Body has been Given an Ego 'I'   83
Five Types of *Pranas* and *Sub-Pranas* in body   85
What happens to *Prana* After Death?   86
Medulla Oblongata and Seven Chakras   87
Reception & Distribution of *Pranas*   89
Sahasrar (the Reservoir of Life Energy)   89
Position of *Nadis & Chakras* in Astral Body   90
Chakras: Aggyia Chakra, Vishuddha Chakra   91-95
    Anahat Chakra, Manipur Chakra, Swadhisthan
    Chakra, Muladhara Chakra

5. Asanas, Exercises, Mudras & Bandhas   97-118
for Awakening The Kundalini

Prayer   99
What are Asanas?   99
Sitting-Posture Asanas for Japa & Meditation   101
Selected Asanas Useful for awakening Kundalini   102-110
    Sarvangasana, Matsyasana (Fish Posture),
    Paschimottan -asana, Ardha-Matsyendra
    Asana, Vajra-Asana, Bhujang-Asana,
    Dhanur-Asana and Marudand-Asana, Shav-
    Asana (Corpse-Asana)
Some Useful Exercises (for Spine):   111-112
    Neck Rotation, Massage of the Scalp &
    Medulla Oblongata, Eyes Rotation Exercises

Useful Instructions for Asanas & Pranayama and   112
   Exercises
Mudras & Bandhas: 112-117
   Mula Bandha, Jalandhara Bandha, Uddiyana Bandha (Nauli Kriya), Maha-Mudra, Maha Bandha, Khechari Mudra, Shakti Chalana Mudra and Jyoti Mudra
Yoga is Equally Important for Women   118

6. Purification of Body, Nadis, Mind and Intellect   119-136

Prayer   121
Purification of Body, Nadis, Mind and Intellect   122
Useful Yoga Practices for Purification of Physical   122-127
   Body: *Dhauti, Basti, Jal-Neti, Nauli, Trataka, Kapalbhati*
Pranayama Exercises: 128
1. Nadi Suddhi (purification of Nadis)   129
2. Sukha Purvaka exercise   129
3. Bhastrika   130
4. Ujjayi   131
5. Suryabhedi   132
6. Plavini   132
7. Pranic Healing (The Secret of Reiki)   133
8. The Distance Pranic Healing (Reiki)   134

7. Techniques of Awakening Kundalini   137-158

Prayer   139
The Necessity of a Spiritual Guru   140
Kundalini Shakti is the Spiritual Energy for   141
   Involution
Relation of Yogi with God   143
What Happens during the Meditation?   144
Concentration is Different from Meditation   145

When and How to Meditate?	147
Meditation Techniques for awakening Kundalini	150
Listening & Meditation on Anahata Sounds	151
(Laya Yoga) or *Surat Shabda* Yoga	
Bhakti-Yoga (Yoga with Devotion Worshiping)	153
The Technique of Kriya Yoga in Brief	154

8. Experiences After Awakening Kundalini 159-196

Prayer	161
Experiences After Awakening of The Kundalini	162
The Symptoms of Awakening the Kundalini	163
Flow of Life Currents After Awakening the Kundalini	167
How an Aspirant should Live After Awakening of Kundalini	169
Misconceptions of Awakening Kundalini by many Authors	170
Eight Major Siddhis after Awakening	175
Many Minor Siddhis (Riddhis)	176
General Precautions to be taken care off After Awakening the Kundalini	179
What happens when the following Chakras are opened?	**180-191**
Muladhara, Swadhisthan, Manipur, Anahata, Vishuddha and Aggyia	
Description of Sahasrara Chakra as observed	190
What happens when the Kundalini Pierces the Sahasrara?	191
Problems of Improper Awakening of Kundalini	196
Does Kundalini Awakening Means Self Realization or the Enlightenment?	196

9. Granthis: the Psychic Knots 197-205

Prayer	198
Granthis: The Psychic Knots	199

Brahma Granthi	200
Vishnu Granthi	201
Rudra Granthi	203
Maha Mrituanjia Mantra	205

10. Shaktipat   206-214

Prayer	207
Initiation of Disciple by Shaktipat	208
Warning About Shaktipat by Quacks	212
Restrictions for Shaktipat	213

11. Important Powerful Mantras   215-226

Prayer	217
Mantras for Awakening the Kundalini	217
The Chanting of Mantras for Worshiping of:	218-221
Brahman, Vishnu, Shiva, Guru, Ma Devi	
Durga, Maha-Laxmi and Ganesha	
Mantras for Pacifying the Effect of Nine Planets	221
Single Mantra for the Worship of Nine Planets	222
Separate Mantras for Nine Planets:	222
Mantras for Sun (Surya), Moon (Chandra),	
Mars (Mangal), Mercury (Buddha), Jupiter	
(Guru), Venus (Shukra), Saturn (Shani), Rahu	
and Ketu.	
Mantras for Peace	223
Mantras for Joy & Bliss	223
Maha Gayatri Mantra, Other Mantras	224
Sri Yantra	225

12. Useful & Important Information   227-232

Evolution of Five Gross Elements from Brahman	228
Dissolution of Five Gross Elements into Brahman	228
Five Basic Pranas	229
The Nine Main Elements in the Living Beings	229

Vital Energies & their Regions Responsible for	229
The Gross Body's Main Elements	230
The Gross Body Elements Produces Further Characteristics	230

God-Realization Foundation (GRF)   231
Aims & Ideals
How to become the member of GRF   232

Glossary	233-250
Bibliography	251-253
Index	254-257

XIV

Word

After the success and appreciation of my first book **"God and Self-Realization"** *(Scientific and Spiritual View)*, published in 2002, many valued readers suggested the need to write on the practical techniques about **"Kundalini & Kriya Yoga"**. This book is based upon my whole life yogic experiences, spiritual studies and blessings of the great saints.

The most of the books available on this subject are neither according to the scriptures, nor concise and nor comprehensive. Some have diverted the main topic and have added too much superfluous information like the details of human anatomy, unlimited description of minor chakras and innumerable nadis in the body. This creates confusion and takes us away from the real goal of Self-Realization. Some have ignored, distorted and twisted the most essential aphorisms of Yama & Niyama and have added their own objectionable views to misguide the innocent readers. Although the subject is very vast, still I have tried my best to be concise and to cover the entire necessary information on the subject, in an easy to understand language with glossary of yogic terms.

"Kundalini & Kriya Yoga" covers both theoretical and practical knowledge in the search of God. It is the journey of soul back to God. It is based upon the Holy Scriptures and the direct experiences of realized saints. All the saints have their variety of subtle divine experiences of awakening of Kundalini.

I am fortunate that I was born in India in a spiritual environment and got the blessings of great saints. India is a country, which has given the greatest gifts like Holy Scriptures, Avataras, so many realized saints many religions to the world. The theoretical & practical knowledge of the great *Vedas and Scriptures* is easily available to the seekers of God in their easy to understand languages in India, but the west is deprived of it. In India aspirants have also an advantage to get the direct, contact, interaction and guidance of the great Gurus in seeking their spiritual path. I am fortunate to have the blessings of the great saints like Sri Paramhansa Yogananda, Sri Amar Jyoti Babaji, Sri Mahavtar Babaji and Sri Sathya Sai Babaji.

I am indebted for the great computer help in typing, editing, designing and in providing the various spiritual ideas and thoughts to my wife Vimla Devi, daughter Jai Shree and son Raju Gupta.

I am thankful for a lot of help, inspiration, guidance and discussion on the related topics in this book from many God-devoted persons like Sh. Ashok Verdhan Dewan, Ex-D. D. E; Mr. & Mrs. Prem Bhandari Head of Third Eye Mission; Sh. R.K. Gupta, Head of National Informatics Centre (NIC) and Dr. Archana Gupta, Sr. Scientist & Addl. Director Council of Scientific & Industrial Research (CSIR).

I can never forget the help of all the persons in the publishing and printing of this book.

20-8-2003 --- **Dharam Vir Mangla**

About the Author

Sh. D.V. Mangla, M.Sc. M.Ed. PGDCA got his masters degrees from university of Delhi. Since his birth he was of scientific bent of mind. He joined his Ph.D. in Mathematics at Delhi University in 1969. Since his childhood he used to study the religious books. He used to discuss about God, *Shastras* and the science with saints and learned people. In 1969 a divine miracle of Sri Sathya Sai Baba transformed his soul, life, philosophy and thinking. He became a perfect theist with a firm faith and conviction in God. He totally surrendered himself to God.

After that he was fully interested in knowing and seeking God. He devoted all his energies in the pursuit of God, spiritual studies and yoga practices. This book is based upon his 36 yrs long practical experience of Asanas, Pranayama & Meditation, learned from various advanced saints in Himalayas and YSS. During 1976-78 he served as lecturer in Mathematics at University of Aden. Since 1996 he is working as the principal of a Sr. Sec. School in Delhi.

The Yogoda Satsanga Society (YSS) of India initiated him in 1989 in 'Kriya Yoga'. He is a scholar of Science, Mathematics, Education, Philosophy and Yoga. He has the ability to correlate the Sciences, *Shastras,* Spiritual Science and God. The book is useful to all categories of men, believers, non-believers and the wavering minds about God. I hope this book will help the "Seekers of the Ultimate Truth" as a complete practical guide at home.

Ashok Vardhan Dewan
Ex-Deputy Director Education J & K

PREFACE

"Kundalini & Kriya Yoga" is a complete, comprehensive practical guide & work-book, which covers in detail all the eight aphorism of Patanjali Yog-Sutras: Yam, Niyama, Asana, Pranayama, Pratyahara, Dharana, Dhyana, Samadhi, Bandhas, Mudras, Granthis, Nadis, Chakras, Siddhis & Riddhis, Mantras, Yantras and the sacred technique of **Kriya-Yoga**.

Due to advancement of culture and education the life of man has become too busy and very fast. Time has become the biggest limitation of man. To remain in the direct company of a self-realized guru at his ashram has become a great limitation. But alternatively, this book will work as an instant search-light to guide the seekers of God, sitting at their homes at their convenient time. If followed properly with devotion the 'Kundalini & Kriya Yoga' will surely help the aspirants to realize God and the Absolute Knowledge. They will be blessed with Joy, Bliss, Peace and may get mystical powers known as *Siddhis* and *Riddhis*.

Now the humanity has become more educated and well civilized. We have begun to ask fascinating and subtle questions like who really we are? From where, we have come to this temporary world? Who has imprisoned us in a wondrous body to act forcibly in this world like a puppet? What will happen after our death? Where will I go after my death? Will I take another birth? What is the real purpose of my life? What is this mysterious universe around us? Who made the scientific laws governing the matter and universe? What is the purpose behind the creation of the universe? What is God? Is it possible to contact God? How to know God and how to contact Him? The present book answers both theoretically and practically to all such eternal quarries of man. The author has explained systematically the subtlest subject in an easy to understand practical way.

We hope this book will be most useful to achieve the sound health free from diseases and spiritual enlightenment by anybody, irrespective of cast, religion, faith, age, sex and guru.

Dr. Archana Gupta
Addl. Director & Scientist 'E'
Council of Sc. & Ind. Research
Govt. of India, PUSA
New Delhi.

R.K. Gupta
Sr. Technical Director & Head
National Informatics Centre (NIC)
Govt. of India, CGO Complex
New Delhi.

How to Use This Book?

- Most of yogic terms have been given in italics. Since these are in Sanskrit or Hindi, the western readers may not be familiar of these. To understand these one should frequently consult the glossary and the miscellaneous chapter given at the end.

- Since this is a practical guide, it is desirable and more useful, if the readers read first the theoretical book "God and Self-Realization" (Scientific & Spiritual View) by the same author. The book "God & Self-Realization" will clear most of your doubts about God and will create a strong devotion for God by knowing a broader concept of God. For a yogi a firm devotion to God is a must.

- Page-wise index has also been given at the end. One may search the pages to understand more about the terms used in this book.

- It will be better if the readers read this book as a clean mind free from all kind of pre-concepts. A regular study of the book in a sequence chapter wise will be more useful. One should not skip the chapters.

- The technique of Kriya Yoga should be practiced only after you deserve or pass the spirituality tests conducted by SRFY, otherwise you may not achieve the final aim.

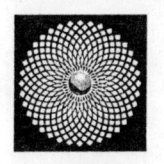

1
Introduction to Yoga

Prayer

What is Yoga?

The Power of the Mind

The Ultimate Aims of Yoga

The Types of Yoga

Yog-Sutras of Maharishi Patanjali:
*Yam, Niyama, Asana, Pranayam,
Pratyahara, Dhyana and Samadhi.*

Types of Samadhies: *Sabhikalpa & Nirvikalpa*

Kundalini Shakti is the Spiritual Energy to
Unite Soul with God (Involution)

Do Not be Afraid of Awakening of Kundalini

Impact of *Maya* can be Removed after
Awakening of the Kundalini

Universe is Just a Great Thought in the Mind of God

So-called Psychology is not a Yogic Science

Only Mental Renunciation is needed by the Aspirants

1
Introduction to Yoga

Prayer

O Divine Mother Kundalini! Thou nature is eternal Bliss & Joy of Brahman. Thou art the cause and the creative energy of Brahman for the manifestation of the Universe. Thou art sleeping and lying dormant as a coiled serpent at the *Muladhara Chakra* of all the human beings irrespective of any cast and religion. Teach me to awaken Thy dormant energy. Teach me to understand Thy great mystery of the spirit, mind, matter, energy and Thy wondrous creative power. Since millenniums and in my numerous past incarnations, I might have forgotten Thee due to Thy strong *Maya*, but I am sure, Thou art have never forgotten me even for an instant. Till now I was busy with Thy enchanting creation and had forgotten Thee. But now I am in search of knowing Thy reality.

O Divine Mother! The Giver of Supreme Knowledge, Absolute Bliss, now wake up! Wake up! Thou art the Beloved of Lord Shiva who is sitting inside the *Sahasrara the thousand–petalled-lotus Chakra*. Do Thou take Thy upward journey to unite with Lord *Shiva* to give Thy children the ultimate knowledge and the self-realization? Reveal Thyself.

What is Yoga?

Yoga is neither a philosophy nor a science. It is much more then ordinary sciences. The sciences provide only little bit information about the creation in the universe. But yoga provides the realization of true knowledge and God. Yogi becomes one with the knowledge. The following questions have confounded humanity since the very beginning. Who am I? Who created the universe? What is the purpose of life & creation? Who gave us a physical body to live in and for what purpose? Can God be seen, contacted, experienced and realized? What is birth, rebirth, death, sleep, dream, meditation and samadhi etc.? Do the saints really achieve the miraculous powers (*Siddhis*) through yoga? Are the miracles realities? If so, how the miracles are performed? The Vedas and the Hindu scriptures undoubtedly antedate all the knowledge of spiritualism in the world. These are the gift of God to humanity. Are these myths, as propagated by some ignorant authors out of their biasedness?

Yoga is a universal divine science and not a religion. It gives answer to all such eternal questions by realizing the truth face to face. Yoga is a system of meditation, mental and physical training that is expected to give knowledge of the supreme reality. Yoga is different from religion and not for a particular society, community or a group of people. It is undoubtedly for all human beings of all religions. It is for the seeking of self-knowledge. One may say yoga is science of verification and realization of true religion of God and the absolute reality of self & creation.

'Kundalini & Kriya Yoga' is a mystic divine science provided to humanity by God through the self-realized saints & Scriptures, by which we can also realize God like the great saints & seers to achieve *Moksha*. Before understanding the Kundalini and its awakening it is important to understand the 'Yoga' and the various *'yogic terms'* used in this book?

Yoga means '**union**' of human soul with the Supreme-Soul or God. The union implies the dualism of both Divine & human spirit. Yoga is the process which librates the human soul from the bondages of *Maya* (attachment to worldly things). There is no other bond stronger than the bond of *Maya*. But there is no other power greater than the yoga & devotion to God to destroy the powerful bond of *Maya*. The union of the soul with God requires the purity of body, mind, spirit and extreme devotion for God. Purity does not mean cleanliness or merely free from sexual impurity, but it is much more. The main exponent of yoga in the world is Maharishi Patanjali.

The Power of the Mind

The purer the mind, free from thoughts, the easier it is to control. Three Gunas mostly control the human mind, which mainly depend upon the nature of food we eat. The food is of three kinds, Satogun, Rajogun and Tamogun. As long as *Rajogun* and *Tamogun* control the mind, it is not possible to bring the mind under our control. An aspirant mainly takes a pure *Satwik* vegetarian food like: milk, dairy products, cereals, pulses, vegetables, juices and fruits etc. and avoids the *Tamsik* food like meat, fish, alcohols and various drugs etc. A *Rajsik* food is allowed casually to everyone.

Emotions like jealousy, envy and animosity agitate mind. The mind can be made peaceful and calm by cultivating the attitudes of indifference towards: sad or happiness, good or bad and success or failure etc. Mind can also be controlled by strong will power, which can be developed only by renouncing the worldly pleasures, desires and attachments. Meditation and strong devotion to God help the aspirants to develop this strong will power.

The enticing advertisements of luxury, comfort and excitement-enthusing consumer goods on television and media conjure up our desire to have them. The joy and happiness from these worldly attachments is temporary and false and not eternal. It is therefore better, not to watch the television too much, but watch it only as a source of necessary information like world-news only. The aspirant should also try to remain unattached to worldly news.

As per the *Taitiriya Upanishad,* the great Rishi Bhirgu aspired to know the ultimate reality. His father god *Varuna (Air)* advised him "Tapas Brahma" (Meditate on Brahma). After prolonged practice, Bhirgu realized that the entire existence came out of a *single universal matter (ether)*, in matter they abide and in matter they dissolve. But his father Varuna did not approved that it was ultimate and advised him to go ahead.

But after some time Bhirgu realized that everything in the universe has come out of the *vital-energy*, sustained by it and again dissolved into it. His father further advised him to go ahead. Later Bhirgu realized that the ultimate reality is the *absolute wisdom*. Meditating further he found that the ultimate reality is *Ananda* (infinite Joy and Bliss). Further Bhirgu searched that the ultimate truth is unfathomable silence and peace beyond description (*Brahman*).

We observe that the ultimate truth depends upon the level and state of our mind. We may come to different conclusions depending on our mind. The ultimate truth is revealed only when the mind is dissolved, since it is the biggest weapon that works under *Maya* to distract us from ultimate truth. *Maya* separates us from God; it goes only if mind is dissolved and peaceful.

An aspirant should also not succumb to the false promises made by the sciences and technologies to eradicate all sorrows from the world. Only the Almighty God can do it. Therefore the aspirant should focus his mind on God, concentrate and meditate upon God all the times. The mind under *Maya* is the cause of ignorance and all the bondages to the material world. The taming of the disturbed mind alone can give the freedom from frequent births and deaths (*Moksha*). The true Ananda comes from within, where God resides in all of us and not from outside which is the *Maya* of God.

The Ultimate Aims of Yoga are

- To get Self-realization
- To become one with God i.e. to merge our tiny spark of soul in the Ocean of God
- To know our ego 'I' and to get rid of it
- To remove our ignorance due to *Maya*
- To get freedom from bondages of births and deaths
- To remain in permanent eternal peace, bliss & joy and to realize the complete ultimate knowledge of everything in the universe
- To understand sleep, dreams, tiredness, happiness etc.
- Many more

To achieve all these aims, the most important thing is your intense devotion and desire to know God & absolute truth, among all your yoga practices. Although all the men & women are eligible and competent for yoga practices, but only very few are able to achieve the ultimate success in one life. This difference is due to the acquired fruits of our past deed and actions (*karmas*) in this and previous lives. A yogi has to first wipe out all the acquired fruits of his past actions good or bad. By the knowledge of the Divine and Kriya yoga practices, a yogi is able to completely wipe out the acquired fruits of past actions and detach his mind from the worldly things. Only after that the Kundalini can be awakened.

Maharishi Patanjali's period is little vague. Many say it is about four hundred years B.C. Many says it is much before. He is a great yogi seer of India has done a great mystical written work on yoga for the benefit of the humanity. He has bifurcated yoga in **eight** necessary steps or aphorisms of *Yog-Sutras*: *Yam, Niyama, Asana, Pranayam, Pratyahara, Dharana, Dhyana (meditation) and Samadhi.*

There is a great misconception about yoga-asanas among most of the beginners, who think that only the *asanas* practice, is yoga. Most of the books on asanas misclaim as book on yoga. It is true that the practice of asanas is very important, to keep our physical body and mind healthy and free from diseases. But the simple practice of different postures or asanas alone has nothing to do with the communion with God, which is the ultimate aim of Yoga.

The *asanas* are enough to most of the persons in the world, who are only concerned to keep their physical body healthy and sound. But *asanas* alone are not enough for the seekers of God. Many persons practice *asanas* regularly, and think themselves as a great yogi. It is a great misconception. *Asanas* are only the third aphorism in the eightfold path of Patanjali *Yog-Sutras*.

Lord Shiva is known as the **Lord of Yogis**. Yoga and Yogis are different terms. The aspirants who practice yoga are called yogis. There cannot be any Yoga without devotion to God. Lord Krishna is known as the **Lord of Yoga**. To illustrate this I would like to tell you the following. In India there are many Yoga organizations in the name of Yoga. Some are providing a free training of *asanas* and *pranayam* to every body, in the open parks every morning. They are doing a great service to look after the health of people. You will find that they provide a beautiful show of group *asanas,* which are useful to keep our body healthy. But most of them ignore devotion to God and simply talk about only the fitness of the physical body to make it free from all kinds of diseases. It is strange that none talked about the devotion and communion with God. What kind of yoga classes are these?

Once some body questioned them for their missing devotion to God. Their reply was strange: "Most of the people are interested only in curing their diseases. They do not come here to seek and commune with God. The members of the organization belong to all the different religions. Some of the members dislike any talk about God. They do not like to prey to God, different from their own religion. So to avoid any confrontation, we have better **shunted out God** from our classes and we do not talk, seek and bother about God for the shake of increasing and pleasing our members."

It is similar in other countries also. In some countries the asana teachers are minting money in the name of Yoga. What type of yoga classes they are teaching, without any talk & devotion to God? Most of the books written by them in the name of "Yoga" are flooded in the bookshops; concerns only with different kinds of a*sana* postures and *pranayama*, as a cure to different diseases are really not the books on Yoga. *For a seeker of God it is better to be alone, than to mix with a crowd without any devotion and concern to God.*

You will appreciate the theme of the following interesting but an imaginary story: "Once a black red-Indian Christian, who was very faithful and devoted to Jesus Christ was forcibly asked to get out from a Catholic Church, by some of the white Christians. The poor black Christian was mentally hurt and suffered with deep sorrow. He was weeping sitting alone outside the Church for a long time. After some time, a strange handsome bearded man came to console him. He was very much loving and sympathetic to him. He asked him the reasons for his sorrows to console him. The black man told him the entire unpleasant incident happened with him. The strange man sympathetically consoled him, "Dear son, do not weep and do not worry any more. I am with you always and I have also been thrown out from this Church." The black-man requested him to tell, who he was? The strange man answered, *"I am the Jesus Christ my son."*

What I want to convey here is, some times we give more importance to our organization and its organized activities but ignore God at the cost of organization. But a real yogi who is the seeker of God is not attached to any organization at the cost of ignoring God. He never forgets his main aim of life to seek God and to know God. He never continues to keep himself attached to an organization, which ignores God and where the devotion to God is missing.

The Types of Yoga

In the ancient Hindu Scriptures there is description of many types of yoga, which are suitable to different types of men depending upon their different natures, abilities, traits & qualities such as: Bhakti (devotional) Yoga, Karma (action) Yoga, Gyan or Sankhya (knowledge) Yoga, Raj (Royal) Yoga, Kriya Yoga (a special type of breathing), Hath Yoga, Kundalini Yoga, Laya Yoga, Mantra Yoga, Tantra Yoga and so many other Yogas.

All the above yogas give more importance to one particular characteristic, nature and practice that is attached to its title. In fact we cannot separate all these yoga practices into the water-tight exclusive compartments. All the human beings have all the characteristics like Devotion, Knowledge & Actions etc., but more or less in different ratios. None of the characteristic is exclusive to other. Some of the aspirants give more importance to asanas, some to meditation, some to knowledge and some to sankirtan (dance in the glory of God) & japa (repetition of the name of the Lord) and others. But it should always be remembered that your intense desire to know God is the most important and common to all yogas.

It is wrong to say that in Bhagwad Gita, Lord Krishna divided the eternal path of yoga into many separate paths like Bhakti, Jnana, Karma and others. There is inherent unity among all these paths. Krishna taught comprehensive spirituality, which is the union of all the yogas through the Bhagwad Gita. Before imparting the knowledge of this eternal knowledge of yoga the Lord said, " It is an ancient yoga. In the beginning He imparted this imperishable yoga to *Vivasvan*, who taught it to Manu and Manu imparted it to *Iksvaku*. Lord also said that He was not declaring any new doctrine but only re-establishing the original eternal verity handed down from master to his pupil."

Generally, Hath Yoga is good to keep the body free from diseases, healthy and to control the Prana. For less educated and more emotional men Bhakti yoga is better. But for highly educated learned men who are generally less emotional, Jnana (knowledge) Yoga is better. Karma Yoga signifies union of God through good works and noble activity. So for the men who are too much involved in worldly activities like business, politics, administration and managements etc. Karma Yoga is better. Raj Yoga or Kriya Yoga involves a high technique of meditation.

It is not proper too say that a particular yoga is better then the other yoga for every body. A yogi automatically follows all the paths of yoga as per his abilities and nature in different ratios. Remember the yoga practice of no two persons is ever same. Even a yoga practice of the disciple is different from his Guru.

But it should always be remembered that the ultimate aim of all yogas is same i.e. self-realization and no self-realization can be achieved before awakening the Kundalini. Samadhi can be achieved only when the Kundalini moves upward crossing the six Chakras. *Bhakti & Karma* yoga leads to *Gyan or Jnana* (Knowledge). *Gyan* Yoga leads to *Bhakti* (devotion) ultimately. As per the Bhagwad Geeta, *Bhakti* and the complete surrender to God is the easiest way among all the yoga practices, but the progress may be little slow. Remember that the Kriya Yoga is the fastest way to achieve the ultimate aim. In Kundalini Yoga we generally concentrate more on the methods of fastest and earliest awakening of the Kundalini.

Yog-Sutras of Maharishi Patanjali

About four hundred years B.C. of Jesus Christ, **Maharishi Patanjali** has given the scientific techniques of yoga and meditation and the **eight** necessary steps of *Yog-Sutras* or aphorisms of Yoga. But do not think that there was no yoga before Patanjali. It was there since the beginning of life. He has defined Yoga as: ***Yogash –Chitvirti - Nirodha***. It means in yoga, *chitvirtis* are to be stopped. *Chitta* is a mental substance. *Chitvirtis* arises from *Chitta* and are the stream of thought-waves or whirlpools in our mind. Countless thought-waves are arising and subsiding from the ocean of Mind. These arises due to the fruits of our past actions (samskaras) and attachments (*vasanas*). If we are able to annihilate and destroy *Chitvirtis* by Yoga practice, our thought-waves in our mind will also be controlled.

Remember that at a particular instant of time we are aware of only about a single thought existing in our mind. We forget the rest of the things of the universe & even about our physical body at that instant of time. We have only one mind and can have only one thought at a particular instant of time, in our mind.

When the mind becomes thoughtless, peaceful, calm, and serene, and cut its connection with the five senses it becomes unaware of the physical body, then it is said to be in the state of **Meditation**. Then the yogi enjoys peace, happiness and bliss. Your real happiness is within you, you can't get it from money, women, children, fame, rank or power.

In the meditation state of consciousness, only the observer or ego 'I' or the self is remained, and everything else vanishes. The observer is situated in its ownself and observes its ownself without using any sense organs. It is a wonderful state of consciousness with ananda, bliss and joy. ... (*Patanjali Yogdarshan: Samadhipad*-I: 2,3,4)

To achieve self-realization faster & without any problem all the *Yog-sutras* are to be followed in an ordered sequence as follows. And no sutra is to be ignored.

1. *Yama:* A yogi should observe his moral code of conduct and restraint himself from its violation. This is known as *Yama*. A yogi must observe the rules like: non-violence, truthfulness, honesty, chastity, non-covetousness, non-acceptance of others possessions. He should love all, help the poor, never over-eat, observe regular fasting and should have the sympathy to sorrowful, poor and deprived etc. Yama and Niyama are the do's and don'ts principles accepted by all the religions.

2. *Niyama:* Observing the personal virtue and disciplining himself by a yogi is known as *Niyama*. Observance of ones religion is known as Niyama. The yogi should develop the good habits like: contentment, purity of thoughts in speech and action, study of scriptures and *Shastras*. Yogi should restraint his worldly desires. Devotion to God is must. A yogi should attend *Satsanga* (the company of saints) and serve the poor and needy people. Man is microcosm. Whatever exists in the macrocosm also exists inside man (microcosm). All the manifestation of universe and the worlds are within man and also within Supreme God.

3. *Asanas:* A yogi should practice regularly different kinds of *yog-asanas* (postures) and some light exercises. These asanas promote and facilitate the flow of life energy in different parts of the body organs. Asanas keeps our body free from diseases, healthy and fit to meditate for a long time. Only a healthy body and healthy mind free from all kinds of diseases and tensions can go to a state of deep meditation. A sick body and sick mind is unable to co-operate with the stress and strain of long meditation.

Mainly the cause of sickness and malfunctioning of some of the organs of the body is due to the lack of life force in some body organ. The proper distribution of the life force is disturbed due to the wrong postures and idleness of the body. By different *asanas*, postures and light exercises we try to send the life force, forcefully in every part of the body, which cures the organ.

There is a great misconception about yoga-asanas among most of the beginners, who think that only the *asanas* practice, is yoga and it is sufficient for awakening the Kundalini. It is true that asanas are very important, to keep our body and mind healthy, and free from diseases. But the simple practice of different postures of asanas alone has nothing to do with God communion, which is the ultimate aim of Yoga. The *asanas* are enough to most of the worldly persons, who are only concerned to keep their physical body healthy and sound. But *asanas* alone are not enough for seekers of God. *Asanas* are only the third step in the eightfold path of Patanjali *Yog-Sutras*.

4. *Pranayam:* The ancient yogis discovered that the cosmic consciousness is intimately linked with breath-mastery. The science of willful control of reception, expense and distribution of the cosmic life energy, through the control of breath is known as *Pranayam*. By pranayama the aspirant is able to dis-connect his mind from his five sense organs and whole of his physical body. It purifies our body, blood, the nervous system, mind and the brain cells. It also purifies our *ethereal body*.

By its regular practice life force begins to flow freely through our *Nadis (Ida, Pingla & Sushumana)*. Our mind becomes free from distracting thoughts. A thoughtless and peaceful mind is must to achieve the deep state of meditation. This is a misconception that air contains prana or life energy. Air does not contain prana, but simply oxygen, Nitrogen, Carbon Dioxide and other gases.

Breathing exercises are also not actually the *pranayama*. The *Prana* is the omnipresent cosmic life energy of God and we receive it through the medulla oblongata. Through proper inhalation and exhalation we control our thoughts, which increase the reception and reduce the expense of prana energy. Through pranayama we can send the life energy forcibly, by our will to any part of our body. The purpose of pranayama must be *Pratyahara*.

5. *Pratyahara*: The withdrawal of our consciousness from the outer physical world and to cut off its connection from five sense telephones from the mind and of the physical body is known as *Pratyahara*. Pratyahara is the regular practice of interiorization of the mind and its withdrawal from the out worldly distracting things and thoughts. Slowly our mind becomes peaceful and turns from extrovert to introvert. Our awareness is turned inward, away from the distraction of the five enchanting senses. The mind turns toward higher inner spiritual states of consciousness. Such a state of higher consciousness is known as *Pratyahara*.

6. *Dharana*: *Dharana* means continuous concentration on a single thought. Thousands of stray unwanted thoughts always distract our mind from our goal. We try to focus or concentrate our mind & awareness on a single thought or an object. It may be a part of our body, or a picture or a thought of God, or sound of Om, or a pure thought or an imagination. By regular practice a yogi is able to fix his mind for a long time on a single object or a thought and turn away all other stray thoughts, which distract his mind. By constant practice of Pratyahara, when mind goes within, it is possible to concentrate upon God.

Many yogis begin to learn the art of concentration, by focusing their mind on a candle flame or a small luminous object. After some time, the yogi closes softly his eyes and tries to visualize the same inside his inner vision. His mind just becomes a peaceful observer or viewer and simply watches the thoughts coming in or going out of the mind. If any stray thought comes to his mind he should let it go away just ignored, without any struggle of his mind. This activity of mind is known as *Dharana*.

7. *Dhyana* (Meditation): If a yogi is in the continuous state of thoughtlessness with awareness for quite some time, he is under meditation. In the state of *Dharana* mind is fixed on a single thought or an object for quite a long time. By a constant practice the yogi tries to get away this single thought, then his *mind becomes peaceful free from all kinds of thoughts and distractions*. But even then the sense of ego 'I' remains in his mind. During the state of meditation (*Dhyana*) the yogi forgets his body, cut off the connection of his sense telephones and the mind awareness; but he knows that he still exists.

Patanjali advises us that a Kriya yogi should meditate upon God and the all-permeating omni sound of Aum. The sound of Aum can be heard first in the body then in the whole universe. All the particles, atoms and molecules are vibrating and oozing out the *Anahat* sound of Aum. It can be heard even by closing the ears.

In this state of consciousness a Kriya yogi does not have the awareness of any space, time and place, but only his ego 'I' remains, to watch & observe his wonderful state of bliss and joy. Everything else melts away. Breathing becomes dead slow. The heartbeat becomes slow. But the yogi is still aware of his ego 'I' known as *Ahankar*. The yogi may listen so many *Anahat* sounds during the meditation state and he may try to concentrate upon them to achieve *samadhi*.

8. *Samadhi:* For a Kriya yogi an intent and constant meditation is necessary for entering into samadhi. When the yogi's ego 'I' merges with God or the transcendence of his soul consciousness with Cosmic Consciousness, it is called *samadhi*. In this state of higher consciousness there are extraordinary subtle experiences of subtle worlds. This is the state of *Ananda* (eternal Bliss & Joy) and yogi is in communion with God. It is so joyful that the yogi wishes to remain in this state forever. He becomes free from all kinds of worldly sorrows & desires. The ignorance of the yogi melts away. The *Ahankar* or ego 'I' merges with God. Just as fire burns a heap of dried leaves, similarly the fire of your intense desire to know God burns all the fruits of your past karmas. A yogi gets intuition (*viveka*) and the real knowledge flashes his mind through *samadhi*.

Types of S*amadhies*:

Samadhi is the highest step explained in the eightfold step by Maharishi Patanjali in his *Yog-Sutras*. There are two types of *Samadhies*. *Sabhikalpa Samadhi* (absorption with fluctuations) and *Nirvikalpa Samadhi* (absorption without any fluctuation). A *samadhi* is attained when the meditator, the process of meditation and the object of meditation become one with God. There are various stages of *Sabhikalpa samadhi* as classified by Patanjali. The intermediate state between the two is called *Asampragyata samadhi* (absorption without awareness).

The **Sabhikalpa Samadhi** is the initial stage of God-communion. In this samadhi the life force is withdrawn from the body and the senses. Mind becomes peaceful, thoughtless & interiorized, but with awareness of ego 'I'. The body just disappears or appears dead. The Yogi is fully aware of his body, which remains in the suspended animation state. The yogi's consciousness merges with the Absolute Cosmic Consciousness of God. Yogi is in the state of Bliss, Joy and Ananda. Yogi gets some subtle experiences. There is no higher super natural knowledge in this kind of samadhi. There are many stages and types of *Sabhikalpa Samadhi*.

A Kriya or a Hath yogi practicing *yogic kriya* may attain various kinds of *siddhies (mystical powers)*. But remember that the *siddhies* are the biggest hindrances in attaining self-realization. A wise yogi always ignores his siddhies and do not hanker after them. In this state a yogi can remain underneath the ground or water for months together. Ascend the path of yoga cautiously. *Siddhies* are the enchanting forms of *Maya* to divert the attention of aspirant from the ultimate goal. *Beware of siddhies attained.*

The **Nirvikalpa Samadhi** (absorption without any fluctuation) is a higher achievement than the *Sabhikalpa Samadhi*. *Nirvikalpa Samadhi* gives us full knowledge of *Brahman and perfect awareness,* which further gives us *Moksha* or Liberation of soul from birth and death. In this state, the mind is attuned to the contemplation of *Brahman* with *Brahman*. *Nirvikalpa Samadhi* is difficult to achieve and can be experienced by only the advanced yogis. The total knowledge of the creation is negligible as compared to the knowledge attained by self-realization.

By continuous practicing of this state of meditation a Hath yogi or a Kriya yogi is able to raise his *Kundalini-Shakti* one day, which is sleeping in dormant state in the lowest part of spine known as *Muladhar Chakra*. After awakening of the *Kundalini-Shakti*, our inner journey or the journey of soul back to God (involution) or the divine romance with God begins.

All the above eight aphorism of Yoga (*Yog-Sutras*) are to be strictly followed by regular practice. If one practice meditation without practicing *Yam, Niyama, Asanas and Pranayam* one may be in trouble and may not get success to achieve *samadhi*. Otherwise if one simply practices asanas & pranayam and ignore *Yama, Niyama* and meditation one will not achieve *samadhi*. One should not skip, some of the steps of aphorism (*sutras*) of yoga to achieve the goal faster. *Devotion and love for God are must for all & for an early success*. Those who practice yoga without any devotion for God may become healthy with some of the mystical powers, but can never commune with God.

Kundalini Shakti is the
Spiritual Energy to unite
Soul with God (Involution)

Most of the religions and saints have referred to the their own experiences and the concepts of Kundalini power and the centers of vital powers known as chakras in human body. On one side Almighty God created *Maya* to separate the creation from Him. On the other side God has also gifted, to man the Kundalini power through which man can again unite with God. Maya separates us from God but yoga and devotion unite us with God. The unity with God is possible only after awakening the Kundalini.

Kundalini is a Sanskrit word meaning "that which is coiled". It also means the "Serpent Power" or the "Serpent Fire". The *Kundalini Shakti* mentioned above is different from primary life force or *Prana Shakti*. It is sleeping in dormant form at the *Muladhar chakra*. It is the Supreme Spiritual Power in the human body and lies coiled and sleeping dormant at the base of the spine until awakened. It is the *Creative Intelligent Force of God*. Kundalini is also the coiled up, dormant, cosmic power that underlies all organic and inorganic matter within us. It is also known as the *'Voice of Silence'*. *Kundalini Shakti* is awakened by regular practice of *Yog-Sutras,* Kriya yoga, intense devotion and grace of God. It is generally experienced to yogis as a coiled snake sleeping in two & half round at *Muladhar Chakra*.

Kundalini is the divine liquid fire that rushes up through the interior of spine known as *Sushumana Nadi* and pierces through the six *Chakras* one by one. Chakras are the internal energy centers in the astral body. *Ida, Pingla and Sushumana* are the three main *Nadis* in our astral body. Without the awakening of *Kundalini* no subtle or *Samadhi* experience is possible. *Kundalini Shakti* is said to be the cosmic force, power or energy of the divine that created the universe and it is constantly evolving and developing new materials, atomic and sub-atomic particles and their different innumerable forms.

Kundalini is the super-intelligent cosmic energy behind consciousness responsible for the involution (journey of soul back to God) of human beings. Generally *Kundalini*

Shakti is spontaneously awakened with the grace of God. If *Kundalini* is awakened without prior purifying of the body, mind and spirit, it may give a great trouble to most of the yogis. Some times its huge mysterious power is uncontrollable by the yogis, as the inner passage of *sushumana* in the spine is not prepared for it. The danger is less if it rushes upward without any blockade in *Sushumana* but more if it turns downwards or sideways.

Do Not be Afraid of Awakening of Kundalini

A Kriya yogi should not be afraid of awakening of his *Kundalini*, if he is practicing and following all the *Yog-Sutras* properly. But before it's awakening, he must purify his body, mind and soul. The process of involution (the journey back to God) and spiritual unfoldment starts only after the awakening of the *Kundalini Shakti*. *Kundalini* is an initiation for entry into the ocean of divine knowledge.

As the *Kundalini* pierces the *Chakras* one by one, there are some subtle inner experiences of subtle worlds to the yogi and he achieves many *siddhies* (divine miraculous powers and knowledge). Self-realization or enlightenment is possible by awakening the *Kundalini Shakti* and rushing up all the *chakras and merging with Lord Shiva in Sahasrar*. A yogi cannot claim himself as spiritual *Guru* without awakening of his *Kundalini Shakti* and raising it upto the *Sahasrar*.

Kundalini Yoga: The yogic practices, which helps faster in the awakening of the *Kundalini* is called Kundalini Yoga. Description of Kundalini is found in the secret teachings of all spiritual literature of most of the religions throughout the world. It is not an exclusive separate yoga from others.

The Impact of *Maya* is Gradually Removed After the Awakening of Kundalini Shakti

Maya is the power of God by which cosmic delusion was created. It is a cosmic force by which *Brahman* has separated Himself from His own creation. The power of super consciousness to separate & divide into many is called *Maya Shakti*. Before the creation of universe, God was alone. When God started the creation, He became the Creator.

As claimed by the scriptures and the self-realized saints our universe is not an ultimate reality, but it is just the God's dream or a thought of His Mind. God is dreaming the dream of cosmic motion pictures on the delusive human consciousness. *Maya* is responsible for the manifestation of 'formless' God to provide different "forms". *Maya* reduces the omni powers of Cosmic Consciousness to limited existence of matter, mind, intelligence and soul. Due to *Maya* we have forgotten that we were God in the beginning and we will again merge in God in future. Due to *Maya* we also feel our association with the body and ego 'I'.

After the awakening of the Kundalini the impact of Maya is gradually removed as the Kundalini rises up and pierces the chakras. Aspirant gets victory over the five gross elements gradually.

The Universe is Just a Great Thought in the Mind of God

The universe is just a great thought in the mind of God. If God just stops His dreaming, the universe will dissolve immediately into God. For a child the motion pictures on television screen appears to be true and real, but the pictures on television screen are only images created by light and nothing more. Similarly the universe is just a motion picture or a dream of God on a four-dimensional screen of space & time by a universal hidden projector.

For a dreaming man the dream appears to be a total reality. The dreaming man forgets every thing of this awakened universe and even the existence of his physical body in this world. Man has the power to dream and create his own dream universe. Similarly this universe is simply a great dream of God and the creatures are just active images or puppets in His Universal Dream.

Maya *is different from an illusion or delusion. Maya cannot be removed by our human intellect and without the grace of God. Maya is the power of God, which creates an illusions and delusions, to* **separate** *the creation from the creator.*

We know fog vanishes before the Sun. Similarly our ignorance due to *Maya* vanishes when the *Kundalini Shakti* rises and crosses the six *Chakras* in the spine. We remove the husk that covers the rice or wheat. Similarly we remove the ignorance, delusion and *Maya* that adheres to the mind of man by the regular practice of Kundalini Yoga. During *samadhi* when *Kundalini Shakti* crosses the chakras one by one, we realize the absolute truth and knowledge face to face and nothing else is needed to explain.

Our two eyes gives us the view of the vast expanse of the universe and space; but our eyes cannot see our own face to which they belong, without a mirror. However the two eyes are the part of our body, the eyes cannot see the back and the inner parts of our body. Even the outer and inner visible parts of our body are not same as visible through the powerful microscopes. Whatever is visible through the naked eye is an illusion or delusion, not the absolute reality. After the awakening of the Kundalini, it rises above in the *sushumana nadi,* crosses the chakras, and then it makes us free from our illusions, delusions and *Maya.*

Our eyes can see but cannot talk or hear. Our tongue can talk but cannot see or hear. Similarly our ears can hear, but cannot talk or see. One sense organ cannot do the work of the other organ. The God and the Divine can be grasped only by awakening of Kundalini through devotion and true *sadhna.* Love and devotion unites us with God, but *Maya* separates us from God. *Maya* completely vanishes only when *Kundalini Sha*kti arises and meets the Lord *Shiva* sitting in *Sahasrar* (thousand petalled) Chakra at top of the skull.

So-called Psychology is Neither the Science of Soul nor the Yogic Science

The word 'Psycho' means Soul, Spirit or Mind. Hence the world 'Psychology' means 'the Science of Soul, Spirit or Mind'. But due to the misconception created by the development of science in the twentieth century, most of the western psychologists stopped believing in the existence of Soul, Spirit or Psycho. Consequently the Psychologists stopped learning about Soul, Spirit and Mind. They limited themselves to study only the external human behavior and ignored the ultimate inner cause of the behavior.

All the modern Psychologists like Freud Sigmund, Jung C.G. and others devoted their life to study only the human behavior, conscious, subconscious, unconscious mind and sex instincts etc, which all are under *Maya*. These Psychologists can be considered simply as Behaviorologists but not as yogis. They were not at all concerned to seek God. To understand the ultimate cause, realm of Soul, Spirit and Mind is beyond the comprehension of these so-called Psychologists of today. Their theories are childish, far from truth and create hindrances in the path of yoga.

No man can realize God, Spirit, Soul and Mind, unless he loves & seek God, day and night, and follows the path of yoga. So for an aspirant, who wants to realize God, it is better for him to avoid the study of the subjects like psychology, which may adulterate his mind. Otherwise it will be difficult for him to wash away the misconceptions created by these subjects. For an aspirant a clean slate like peaceful mind without any thought is better than a mind full of billions of unwanted thoughts and worldly learning.

I advise to read only the *Scriptures* and the literature of the saints, saviors and those who have really devoted their life in the pursuit of God. Ignore the literature and the ideas of worldly people unconcerned to God.

Only Mental Renunciation and Not the Sanyias is needed by an Aspirant

As per the Scriptures and Bhagwat Geeta it is sufficient to *renounce only mentally* the worldly things and doesn't need to leave actually his wealth, family and friends. A householder or a king has the same right to seek and to know God as a *sanyasi,* but it may be little more difficult for him as he has to fulfill all responsibilities of his family along with God. Hence a yogi needs not to leave his family to become a *sanyasi* to seek & know God.

A yogi or an aspirant is generally said to renounce the worldly things, desires, sex, physical pleasures, wealth, fame and family etc. But it is wrong to presume that he doesn't want to achieve anything. The truth is just opposite. By sacrificing all worldly things a yogi want to achieve God, who is the giver of everything in the world. In fact a yogi want to achieve everything in the universe by simply renouncing the petty worldly things, which are like toys, dolls and toffees, provided by *Mother Maya* to keep Her kids busy in their playing and make Her free to complete the important works.

Remember a yogi wants to achieve everything in the universe by sacrificing petty little things, but a *bhogi* (worldly man) is satisfied with the little petty worldly things and sacrifices God who is the giver of everything. So a *bhogi* sacrifices everything in lieu of petty things is more renounced person than a yogi. Is it not so?

Remember: "Our proud of little learning and sallow knowledge is our biggest enemy and a dangerous virus to learn more and to know the absolute reality of the universe. Through the science whatever we have learnt or learning is only about the creation. It is just a glimpse of the dream of God, which provides us a little information. The whole universe and all the creatures are the images or puppets on a 4-dimentional screen of space and time, projected by a universal stereoscopic holographic hidden projector in the mind of God. Due to Maya, we are misinterpreting the dream images as the reality, which is false."

! Om Peace, Peace, Peace!

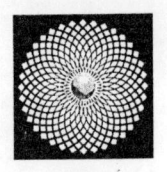

2

The Basic Concepts of Kundalini Yoga

Prayer
The Theory of Kundalini and Kriya Yoga
Life Energy is Different from Physical Energies
What about Tibetan Buddhism?
Did Tibetans know about Kundalini?
Physical Body is not as it looks to our Senses
The bodies of men and other living beings
    are the biggest chemical industries.
Physical & Mental Works are Different
Do not Over-eat but must Do Regular Exercises
Many Prohibitions for an Aspirant
What are Granthis?
How to Increase the Reception and Retention of Life Force?
Vegetarian Food is Full of Life-Energy
Devotion & Love for God is Must
Never Forget God
What are Om & Anahat Sounds? What is Laya Yoga?
Harmony with Nature And Becoming One with All
Harmony with The Five Gross Elements of Creation
Possession of a Human Soul by some other Soul

2
The Basic Concepts of Kundalini Yoga

Prayer

O Cosmic Mother Divine! O Divine Creative Energy! Thou art hidden in all the human beings. Thou hast manifested as *Prana* the life force, magnetism, electricity, sound, gravitation cohesion, adhesion, nuclear and all types of physical energies. Thou art the ether in which the universe rests in Thy bosom. We bow to Thee, O Mother of all worlds. Thousands of suns, stars & galaxies do shine on thy beauteous bosom.

As per the Holy Scriptures, Thou art the Holy Ma Durga, Maha-Laxmi, Maha-Saraswati, Ma Kali, Adi-Shakti, Tripura-Sundari and Raj-Rajeswari. Thou hast manifested all the forms.

O Mother Kundalini! Now wake up! Purify and open the Sushumana Nadi, take the path of the Chakras to Sahasrar, merge in Thy consort Lord Shiva and reveal Thy Absolute Reality.

The Theory of Kundalini Yoga

Kundalini means circular coil like that of *'serpent'*. That is why the word 'serpent' is associated with it. A serpent is powerful with its fangs and poison. Those who know, how to tame serpent power, can tame the serpent. Serpents live hidden inside earth and behind bushes under the ground. Kundalini is latent and dormant vital force in human body, resides at *Muladhara*. When aroused it pierces various *chakras* and unites with Lord Shiva in *Sahasrara* which leads to self-realization. Thou art do not belong to our physical, astral or mental plane and cannot be found there by the doctors, scientists and psychologists. Thou art belongs to a still higher causal plane, which is beyond the concept of matter, time and space (beyond the Relativity of Einstein).

The individual Kundalini energy hidden in humans is an infinitesimal part of the divine cosmic Kundalini energy. It enters the embryo along with the soul soon after conception. After completing the assigned task of creating the body of the baby in the womb, it lies dormant in the coiled shape and hence the name Kundalini. The individual Kundalini is just fraction of the divine cosmic energy, which pervades cosmos and is said to be effulgence of spiritual energy of the Absolute Brahman. The individual Kundalini energy of each man is different from that of other.

Kundalini can be awakened by *Pranayama, Asanas and Mudras by Hath Yogis*; by deep concentration and training of mind by Raj-Yoga or Kriya-Yoga; by extreme devotion and perfect self-surrender by emotional men (*Bhaktas*); by analytical will, thinking & analysis by the knowledgeable aspirants (*Jnanis*); by Mantras & Tantra by *Tantriks*; and by the grace of Guru as *Shaktipata*. No samadhi is possible without awakening of the Kundalini and no self-realization or *Mukti* is possible without merging of Kundalini with Lord Shiva in Sahasrara.

Generally a real Guru has inner divine insight (*Viveka*) to know the inner achievements of his disciples. He is capable of right & proper advise for the earliest awakening of their Kundalini as a qualified doctor is capable of rightly prescribing the suitable medicine and treatment to his patients. Only one kind of medicine is generally not suitable equally to all the patients. Similarly one kind of yoga-practice is not equally suitable to all the aspirants of different nature. So a real guru is capable to decide a better path of yoga for an early success.

A yogi mainly concentrates to awaken his Kundalini at the earliest through the purification of his body, mind and spirit, through special postures (*asanas*), *pranayama (controlling life-force through breath control), bandhas, mudras, sat-karmas, and meditation.* He mainly concentrates on the *Anahat* inner sounds known as *Laya* yoga. The Kundalini yoga is mainly Hath yoga and *Laya* yoga. It gives bliss, joy and liberation to soul.

The unseen life force (*prana*) is subtle, hidden and difficult to control. It governs our physical body automatically. It is received through Medulla Oblongata, distributed in the body through Aggyia chakra and other chakras. The prana is flowing *downward* in the spine, outgoing into the sex organs, through a coiled passage at the base of the spine in the coccyx known as Kundalini sleeping in Muladhara. This outgoing life force stimulates the sex instinct, unites male & female, and is utilized or wasted in sexual activity. The symbol of snake represents its nature, which is powerful and poisonous. You can know God only if you conquer your sex power.

An ordinary person does not know the cause of his over sex desire and its related problems, which are due to this outgoing energy. So it is important to observe celibacy and to control the sex instinct by an aspirant. Some of the ignorant writers are propagating opposite to it. For them the moral and sex ethics and values have no meaning. According to them there is no eligibility criteria for a yogi for the awakening of his Kundalini through *Shaktipat*. But remember the awakening of Kundalini of an undeserving man may create uncontrollable problems.

The aspirants should try to stop this wastage of life energy and redirect its flow back from Muladhara to Medulla Oblongata and brain. This mystic force unites the soul with the almighty God. The aspirants learn how to withdraw the entire life force that moves through the six spinal chakras, senses and sex organs to flow backward to Sahasrara. The coiled Kundalini life current when awakened produces a remarkable spiritual and physical sensation in the body. It provides an absolute mastery over the senses and sex instincts.

During our awakened state of mind, there is too much utilization of life-energy in all the five senses, digestive system, nervous system, and in heart palpitation etc. During meditation we withdraw life energy from the senses, stomach, heart and other parts of the body. The digestion by stomach becomes slow and it is kept empty, the heart palpitation becomes very slow and breathing is slow. During meditation the expense of life energy is negligible and the aspirant tries to force the life energy to go up through the Sushumana nadi back to Medulla oblongata and brain. The awakening of Kundalini is done by withdrawing of the life current from the five senses and directing it forcibly into Sushumana. The advanced yogis can consciously take their soul through the Sushumana nadi at any time or at the time of their death. This provides *Moksha* to soul.

We know that the energy polarizes itself into two forms i.e. *potential (static) & dynamic.* There is a static background behind all the activities. Similarly behind all the dynamic activities in the body there is a static centre known as *Muladhara Chakra,* where the serpent Kundalini power is sleeping or stored in static potential form. This dormant potential Kundalini is awakened and activated by pranayama and other yoga practices and it becomes dynamic. Then it rushes up into the *Sushumana Nadi* and pierces the six chakras in its path. Lastly it unites with Lord Shiva in *Sahasrara* (thousand patelled lotus). This union is the self-realization i.e. soul merges with God. It gives *Moksha* or liberation to the soul. It is also known as Christ or Krishna or Cosmic Consciousness of the soul.

When the Kundalini sleeps, its static power sustains the world consciousness. But when it is awakened the yogi loses all consciousness of the world. He enters into causal world and passes into the formless universal consciousness. Yogi loses his physical body consciousness and enters into his causal body. When the Kundalini wakes up the yogi apparently sleeps for the world and loses his body consciousness. He goes to Samadhi state, which reveals the secrets of spiritual forces and God.

The Cosmic Power is known as *Maha-Kundalini Shakti.* It is dynamic and works collectively throughout the universe, while individual Kundalini Shakti works in the body of a particular man and is at rest. A living human body is a microcosm and the whole universe is macrocosm. This personal form of Kundalini is responsible for the creation of the individual. In the biological process of development of the fetus in the mother's womb, the head and brain are formed first. Next, the spinal cord is formed from the nerves that branch from the brain, and the trunk is formed. Then the other organs like the hands, and the feet are formed. The totality of the nerve centers in the brain is referred to as the *Sahasrar chakra*. This is the cause of the process of creation.

The outgoing currents of life energy stimulate the nerves of creative sex force. It tempted the physical union in male & female, whereby they lost divine consciousness at the cost of sex. We cannot blame that the Kundalini Shakti is responsible for our attachment to the material world and sex instincts, as we cannot blame that the blasting explosive chemicals like RDX & Dynamite in bombs is responsible for the destruction activity of the terrorists through its use.

As per *Swami Satyananda Saraswati*, "the awakening of the Kundalini causes a transformation and transcendence in life of an aspirant. He experiences the visions of God and the higher realms of truth. There are subtle changes in his mind, mood, priorities, desires and worldly attachments. The fruits of past karmas begin to be washed away. All the body cells are fully charged with the life energy and the process of rejuvenation begins. The physical, mental, emotional and the spiritual involution (journey back to God) begin to take place. "Once the great *Shakti* (power) awakens, man is no longer a gross physical body operating with a lower mind and a low voltage *prana* (quantum cosmic energy). Instead every cell of his body is charged with the high-voltage *prana* of Kundalini. And when total awakening occurs, man becomes a junior god, an embodiment of divinity."

The Old Testament's symbol of Kundalini shown in this picture is significant in Christianity when Christ suggests Kundalini awakening as the true destiny of all Christians: *"And as Moses lifted up the serpent in the wilderness, even as the son of man be lifted up: That whosoever believeth in him should not perish but have eternal life"*

God told Moses "make thee a serpent, and set it upon a pole: and it shall come to pass, that everyone that is bitten, when he looketh upon it, shall live. And Moses made a serpent of brass, and put it on a pole, and it came to pass, that if a fiery serpent had bitten any man, when he beheld the serpent of brass, he lived"

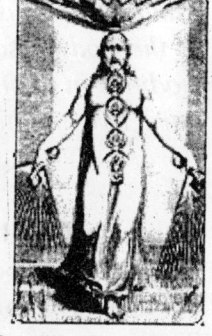

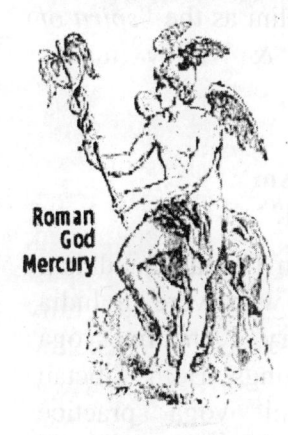

The symbol of Kundalini in this picture in the hands of Roman God Mercury confirms that Christianity also had the concept of Kundalini. They called it a reflection of the Holy Ghost, and worshipped its manifestation during the Pentecost reunion.

Mercury said that *'The Holy Spirit is My Mother'*. *'The Kingdom of God is within you'* (Luke 17:21).

Famous Psychologist Dr. C.G. Jung a student of Sigmund Freud and Esther Harding believed in a "Higher Unifying Centre" for the superconscious and for the life of the individual as a whole. He called this centre as 'Transpersonal or Higher Self'. The spiritual unfoldment may give experiences of the superconscious realms and the aware of the

Ego 'I' self. The process is known as Self-Realization, which leads to the identification of 'I' with the Higher Self."

"Kundalini is one of the greatest energies. The whole body of an aspirant starts glowing because of the rising of the Kundalini in Sushumana. Because of this, unwanted impurities in the body disappear. The body of the aspirant is suddenly modifies in appropriate proportion and the eyes look bright & attractive and his eyeballs glow."

... Sant Gyaneshwara, 1275 AD, Gyaneshwari, Ch.VI

Although **Buddha** did not believed in God as he was always silent about God, but spoke of the *"middle path"* to achieve nirvana. By 'middle path' he actually mean the central Sushumana Nadi, through which the Kundalini ascends after awakening. Lao Tze also described Kundalini as the *"spirit of the valley"*. Spirit means Kundalini & valley means Sushumana Nadi.

Did Tibetans or Buddhism Knew about Kundalini?

The *Natha* and *Vajrayana* religious sects in Tibetan Buddhism took their origin from the *Mahasiddhas* who were in India from the 8th century to the 12th century. Kundalini yoga practices formed the core of their teachings. Both Tibetan Buddhist and contemporary Kundalini yoga practice Kundalini yoga. It was spoken of as 'Candali yoga' and was known as 'gTummornal', 'byor' in Tibet. Candali yoga was the main practice of the famous Tibetan yogin Milarepa.

There are many other spiritual paths of practice, such as *Zen, Jainism, Preksha* and *Vipasana* meditation. It is strange that they believe in the existence of *soul* but not in the *Supreme Soul (God)*. According to them, Kundalini is irrelevant. Their yogic paths concern only with the health and the physical body, but ignore God intentionally. Such practitioners and their preachers have neither been able to awaken their own Kundalini nor got any experience of self-realization. Even the slightest experience of God is enough to believe in God for the rest of life. It is not clear, without any enlightenment & the union of soul with God, what kind of yoga (union) they claim? On whom they meditate? When the *Jainism* do not believe in the existence of *Bhagwan* (God) and His incarnations, how do it claim, *Mahavir* as *Bhagwan-Mahavir*? This is contradictory and confusing.

The Chinese '*qi gong*' practitioners have reported their identical yogic experiences, similar to those of Kundalini yoga aspirants and believe in Kundalini Shakti.

Life Energy is Different from the Physical Energies

'*Prana*' is a Sanskrit word. It means 'life energy'. The life energy controls the whole universe including all the livings, non-livings and inert matter. It is a wondrous kind of cosmic energy and has infinite intelligence too. The other physical energies like heat, light, sound, magnetism, electricity, nuclear and mechanical etc. are inert without any intelligence. Since the physical energies have no intelligence, these cannot think and decide to work or not to work or how to work? To understand clearly the life energy first try to understand the following concepts:

Physical Body is not like as it Looks to Our Senses

Our Physical body consists of five sense organs, five work organs, digestive system, excretion system, nervous system, blood circulatory system, spine and brain and so many other organs. All these systems are interdependent and interconnected with each other in a perfect network of cells. Understand that each of the body organs is further made up of billions of tiny living cells. The cells in each organ are well organized and arranged in a systematic beautiful design and in a network, which comprise our flesh and bones. Further all the organs are well arranged in a well organized network and working in perfect co-operation with each other to form the physical body of different shapes. *Remember a human body consists of nearly twenty eight thousand billion cells of many kinds, well connected in a network.* Our ordinary commonsense does not inform all these.

All the cells are further made up of so many complex chemicals, molecules and whirling atoms all in motion. None of the atom or molecule is at rest. Each cell is composed of complex chemicals, proteins, genes, RNA & DNA molecules etc. Miraculously the atoms and molecules are dancing and vibrating in circular motions at a very high speed without colliding with each other in infinitesimal closeness to each other.

The atoms are further composed of electrons, protons, neutrons and so many other elementary particles. The elementary particles are nothing but *tiny sparks of thought* in the Mind of God. These particles are further arranged in each cell and further these cells are arranged in the physical body. These arrangements need infinite intelligence of God. No inert physical energy can make the arrangement of these cells since it requires intelligence. *Hence it is clearly evident that infinite intelligent life energy is doing all kind of arrangements, networking and fine works. The whole universe is fully controlled by the Infinite Intelligence of God.*

The Bodies of Men and other Living Beings are the Biggest Chemical Industries.

To design, install and run such a huge chemical industry with an infinite intelligent network, running inside man and other living beings, *the whole surface of earth is not sufficient*. It is impossible for the engineers to design it in such a small compact body, which does not need any worker and quality control and management people inside the body.

All the human body organs are constantly working in perfect co-operation in a network, continuously day and night. It requires an intelligent energy to run and manage it in the small compact physical body. This huge factory inside the human body is not affected, whether we take food or not. The food and fluid we take in, simply supply heat, electrical, chemical and mechanical inert energies and a few complex chemicals the body needs. If we stop taking food at all, all our body organs and systems like heart, sense organs, brain, digestive system, excretion system and nerves systems etc. will still continue to work as usual till our death. None of the body system stops working due to the lack of food energy. But all the body organs stop functioning instantaneously just after our death when the life force leaves our body. It is just as the electric powerhouse is switched off and every thing comes to stand still instantly.

*It clearly shows that the body is not running by food alone, but it is working due to some infinite intelligent energy known as **life energy** or the prana.* Strength comes from within, not from the muscles alone. Life of a human body is sustained from our power within. It does not depend solely on food.

Brain is Different From our Mind

The brain is a physical organ of our body and the mind is a cosmic energy, which works on brain to do the mental work. There is only one mind energy throughout the universe, which works in different brains of all the living beings. It is just like the same electrical energy, which works in millions of electrical equipments throughout the country.

The brain requires the omnipresent cosmic mind energy to function its different faculties. Remember that **Mind is not the brain**. A doctor can do the operation of a brain, but not of the mind. Mind is not a physical thing, but brain is. Mind is a cosmic energy of God & it functions on brain when the body is alive. It is true that we are tired after both the physical and mental works. Physical energy is required to do the physical work and is supplied by food (chemicals & nutrients etc.). But the mind energy and the life force comes from cosmos. By doing a mental work not much food or chemical energy is consumed or required, and only the life force and mind energy are used. *So the person doing only mental work should not overeat when he is tired, rather he should do regular exercises to consume the surplus calories supplied by the food.*

We Must Not Over-Eat & Do the Regular Exercises

So it is important and necessary to *take less food and do some exercises or asanas* daily and regularly for the persons who are always busy to do some kind of mental work in their offices or work places. Because due to the lesser physical work the amount of calories or energy supplied by the food they have taken in, is not consumed properly by their body. When people get tired after their mental work they usually take rest instead of doing some exercises or physical work. A mentally tired person should not think that his body should take physical rest and consume more rich food to get rid of the

The Basic Concepts of Kundalini Yoga

tiredness. This is a delusion and cause of their overeating, overweight and disfiguring of their body. Hence the persons doing mainly the physical work require more rich food to supply the extra physical energy and chemicals they consume.

It is a misconception that thousands of our body organs like heart, stomach, kidneys, sense organs and so many glands are functioning due to the energy supplied by the food. The food mainly supplies the heat, chemical and mechanical energy to do the physical work by living creatures. The entire body organs functions regularly, even if we stop taking any food, till death of the body. The scientists still does not know exactly by which energy all the body organs are functioning. None of the body organ including the sense organs & brain can function without some kind of energy. Remember, the entire body organs function due to life-force received by the medulla oblongata & not due to the energy supplied by food or breathing.

Food plays a prominent place in yoga. A yogi should take only moderate *satwik* vegetarian diet mainly fruits, vegetables, almond and plenty of milk. He must avoid eating meat, fish, alcohol, drugs, tobacco, garlic, onions, unripe or overripe fruits and all other *tamsik* foods.

The prohibited diets create hindrances, causes many diseases and problems after awakening of the Kundalini. All the efforts of an aspirant may go waist if it is not followed. However the *Rajsic*-foods are allowed, if taken rarely on some occasions.

Many Prohibitions for an Aspirant

As per the Holy *Shastras* there are so many prohibitions for an aspirant. A yogi must follow strictly the *Yama & Niyama* as defined in the *Scriptures* and not as per some of the western authors. Most of the western authors on yoga and the related subject have a shallow knowledge of Hindu *Scriptures*. Many of them have no clear knowledge of this subject. Most of them have been grown up in a modern & western style of life i.e. eat, drink & be marry. Most of the western philosophies are concerned only to how to enjoy and live well. On the other hand the Hindu Philosophy is concerned both on how to live well and how to die well.

Some of the authors, philosophers and intellectuals are moody, moderate and proud of their bookish knowledge. They do not give importance to the values attached to character, moral, sex and temptations. It is difficult for them to follow the *Yama & Niyama* as defined by the Vedic Scriptures. They have been brought up in an environment contradictory to *Yama & Niyama*. So instead of correcting and molding themselves, they generally try to justify their own acquired wrong habits through their ill-logics. They try to convince their readers to remain the same. The readers should not accept it.

Such authors have only a little bookish knowledge of yoga gathered from here and there. They are unable to follow and understand the *Vedic Shastras, which* are originally in *Sanskrit* or in Indian languages. Most of them did not get the opportunity and the company of the great Indian yogis and saints. Like the Ashrams in India, many of them have also opened their own yoga schools in their countries. Interestingly these schools are providing training only for asanas and pranayams. They are ignoring the other six aphorisms of yoga. They are misguiding the real seekers of God and are minting money too. The books written by them are generally rubbish inter-mixed with their personal modern-western thoughts. A real seeker should avoid such adulterated Yama & Niyama.

For example: These authors do not understand the difference between: the ordinary love; love between mother-child; Love & devotion to God and the sexual-love instinct like animals. They simply understand that love means sex and the Kundalini Shakti is also a sex power. Interestingly, if the sex instinct of some one is aroused they presume it as his awakening of the Kundalini.

They are of the opinion that there is no harm in violating the Yama & Niyama prescribed in the scriptures like: frequent over-sex, polygamy or sex with many; habitual of drugs, alcohol, wine, smoking, eating meat, fish, eggs, *tamsik* food & violence against the living beings etc. They propagate that the worldly attachments and desires have nothing to do with yoga. Instead of strictly following the *Yama & Niyama*, they are changing the *Yama & Niyama* itself, as per their sweet will and to please their readers too. They are also misinterpreting and adulterating the facts mentioned in the *Holy Shastras*. It is advisable for a seeker of God not to read the adulterated literature of such authors.

A yogi must control his sex instinct and worldly desires through his inner strength of will and deep meditation. The seeker must avoid sex with other then the spouse. The Seeker of God should avoid taking meat, fish, eggs, drugs, alcohol, wine, and smoking. He should try to be a pure vegetarian and should not over-indulge in worldly activities. He should avoid the company of the people unconcerned to God and who have no faith in Holy Scriptures.

In nut cell a seeker of God should **avoid** the following:
1. Sex other than spouse and remain faithful to spouse.
2. Control, balance and minimize the sex instincts.
3. Drinking wine and all kinds of alcohols.
4. Smoking and drugs.

5. Eat meat, fish, eggs & other non-vegetarian foods.
6. Over-indulging in worldly activities.
7. Too much reading of newspapers, over viewing of TV & other media.
8. Dirty politics without principles.
9. Company of people unconcerned with God.
10. Over indulgence in business or administrative jobs.
11. Highly responsible time bound jobs, which creates the tension of completion of work.

What are Granthis?
(The Psychic Knots)

Granthis are the Psychic knots of the nerves in the spinal Chord made up of subtle matter. They play an important role in the awakening of the Kundalini, partially or fully. There are three major Granthis: *Brahma Granthi, Vishnu Granthi and Rudra Granthi.* Brahma, Vishnu & Rudra (Mahesha) are the Trinity of God as per Scriptures. These Granthis are the main hindrance in the movement of the Kundalini energy upward. So along with the opening of the six Chakras, the Granthis are also to be opened.

How to Increase our Reception and Retention of the Life Force?

During the day in the *awakening state* of consciousness (when mind is not tuned) the reception of the life force is less and the consumption is more. *During awakening* state life energy is used in digestion, blood circulation, in sense organs, excretion and even in thinking too. Hence till night our body cells are exhausted of their charged life energy, and they need further re-charging by the life energy. *Remember due to the exhaustion of life force in the cells, we feel drowsy and it is also the cause of our tiredness.*

The Basic Concepts of Kundalini Yoga 47

But *during the sleep at night* the function of all our body organs becomes very slow. The connection of our sense organs or sense telephones is cut off from the brain. The beats or pumping of heart and the digestive system becomes dead slow. So the expense of life energy in different body organs becomes negligible. But during sleep the reception of the life force by the Medulla oblongata becomes very high. Our mind is more tuned & is nearer to God, who is the ocean of the life energy. So our body cells get re-charged again during night sleep. Further *during the deep sleep,* our soul is still *more nearer* to God and the reception of life energy becomes many folds. This is the reason why we are fresher in the morning after enjoying the deep sleep instead of the disturbed night. During a *disturbed night,* which is generally full of dreams, we are less tuned with God and the reception of life energy is low.

During the *deep meditation* we are perfectly tuned with God and there is a *resonance* of reception of life energy. The reception is thousands of time more, then the awakening state. Our sense telephones are cut off from our body and the brain. Hence a yogi who practice deep meditation, either need no sleep or a short sleep for few hours is enough for him. Such yogis are less tired and need less rest. Their intuitive & thinking power increases manifold tremendously.

Among the so many body systems the *digestive system* consumes the maximum amount of the life energy. It requires nearly 25% of the total life-energy received. The instant we put any food in the stomach, whether the body needs it or not the digestive system begins to work. It keeps pending all the other important works of the body. Otherwise the body will become sick immediately, if it stops digesting.

But whenever the life-energy is free from the digestion, then 25% of this important life-energy is saved. Then it is available to do more important works, like the repairing of the injuries in the body, fighting with the bacteria of diseases, cleaning of the digestive system and the blood circulatory system and so many other important works. We all know whenever our body falls sick, our hunger gets automatically reduced to save the expense of the life energy and we need bed rest. The nature warns us not to eat much to save the life energy from digestion. That is why during our sickness, we should eat the minimum. The fluids are easily digested and keep the life energy free from digestion, and to fight against the disease. Very soon the doctors will realize this truth.

Hence remember a *weekly fast, limited food and no overeating is the essential requirement for maintaining a healthy body free from diseases.* There have been so many **non-eating saints** in the world from time to time to further affirm this.

Brahmacharya (celibacy) is an important step to save the waste of life-energy. Maximum amount of life-energy is wasted outwardly in the form of semen produced in the sex activity. The energy saved helps to produce the necessary environment to awaken the Kundalini Shakti. It is misleading to say that sex or over-sex has nothing to do with the awakening of the Kundalini. Celibacy is essential for attaining the deep meditation. Karl Jung and Fried might have done some experiments in the field of brain and sex, but they are thousands of mile away from awakening Kundalini, spiritualism and God. In their whole life they could not understand even the basics of soul and yoga.

If a society or culture permits free sex, it will perish like the culture of Rome and Greece. By the observance of celibacy vigor is gained. Excessive loss of semen spreads disease and

The Basic Concepts of Kundalini Yoga

disaster in the body. If a man violates Brahmacharya (celibacy) the law of nature, then he is surely punished by the Mother Nature.

Vegetarian Food is Full of Life-Energy

Food contains only a limited supply of life energy. A vegetarian food like the fresh milk, vegetables, fruits and pulses contain some amount of life-energy. The vegetarian foods are generally the things from vegetation including milk and contain all the five sub-*pranas*. But a non-vegetarian food comes from dead creatures which contains only one life force i.e. *Udana* sub-*prana*, which destroys the body after death. The other four types of life forces (*sub-pranas*) left the dead bodies i.e. all kinds of meat.

We observe that only a small portion of a vegetarian thing is spoiled, if infected by the bacterias or germs. The infected portion can be removed easily from it, as it is generally visible through eyes. But a non-vegetarian food is completely infected by the harmful bacterias & germs throughout the dead body and is not visible through the bare eyes or our senses. The infection of a non-vegetarian food is neither traceable nor can be removed.

It is totally false and a misconception, if we eat meat or blood it will directly go to our muscles & blood. Remember not even a single atom or molecule can directly go inside our inner body, unless & until it is fully digested by our digestive system. The vegetarian foods are generally much easier to digest then the non-vegetarian foods. Therefore our body gets more out of a vegetarian food then a non-vegetarian food.

A non-vegetarian food is of *tamsik* nature. But a vegetarian food is of *satwik* nature. The food served rich in proteins and fat in parties & marriages is a r*ajsic* in nature. *So a yogi should avoid eating the non-vegetarian food and seldomly take the rajsik food to achieve early success by fewer efforts.* There have been some non-eating saints in the world who never ate or drunk any thing in their lives.

Hence, learn the art of **Pranayama** i.e. the techniques of charging our body with life energy. Learn to control the life energy at our will and then we can achieve an excellent health, mental power, victory over diseases and many other important things. This is possible only through the science of *yoga*.

The Holy *Shastras* says that God is beyond the comprehension of mind and senses. Unless we detach our mind from the senses and make the mind peaceful without any thought of distraction, we cannot know God. God is knowable not by our intelligence, but through the intuitive perception in man. **Intuition** is beyond the five senses. Intuition can comprehend the facts, which are beyond the five physical senses. Intuition is the sixth sense of all knowing faculty of soul. By continuous and regular meditation, we have to increase our power of intuition and make the mind peaceful.

Devotion and Love for God are Must for the Seeker of God

During the meditation your devotion & love for God is essential. The spark of this love of God is expressed in all the living beings through us. Understand that the sexual love is different from the devotional love for God. Sexual love is an animal biological instinct, temporary, selfish and a lust for opposite sex. Without this sex instinct there cannot be a sexual love. So we must realize the eternal love for God. This is without any sex instinct, so great and so joyful, but permanent.

The greatest romance that our soul can have is the romance with the Supreme Soul (God). We have no experience and the idea of this divine romance with Supreme-Lover. But once we commune with God, we will find God everywhere. We will realize that everything in the universe is nothing but the manifestation of God. In samadhi or deep meditation God comes, whispers, guides, plays, loves and communicate with us. We are the best creation in the universe and the children of God. God loves all His children good or bad.

Remember, God does not need any thing from us, except our devotion and love to Him. Since our creation, He is also seeking and waiting for our love too. God too suffers when we deprive Him from our devotion & love. We should always devote a little bit of our daily time, to sit alone, to meditate and have a romance with God. Sri Radha[1], Sri Meera, *Gopies,* Sri Chataniya Mahaprabhu, Sri Soor Das and so many other saints are the finest examples of the great divine romance with Lord Krishna.

God is the nearest of the near and dearest of the dear in this crowded illusion-world. We must cry for the love of God as a kid cry for his mother and a miser loves his money. Not even a single breath should go without our devotion to God. When a minimum intrinsic or escape energy of our love and devotion for God is achieved, God comes and reveals to us. Only our intense pure devotion & love can commune and imprison God, nothing else. A yogi should develop an intense fire of pure love for God in his heart. You should always affirm that the beloved God is always with you in your heart, while you are

---

[1] All the lady saints, deities and gods are prefixed with Sri and not Smt.

working, sleeping, dreaming, meditating or doing any other work or activity.

The perishable world is a big stage of divine drama for God. God has given only to man (others not) the freedom to act (good or bad). Our love is the only thing that God does not possess. Only our love can bind God in our heart. Although God is also seeking for our love, but He will never force us to love Him back. We have the freedom to love God or not. But believe me that God is watching, observing and recording all our actions, even our thoughts every moment. *God enjoy all our good actions but also suffers due to our bad actions or bad karmas.* Feel the divine love of God in all human being & other creatures, and carry forward the message of love, peace and service to all.

It is only by the grace of God that one meets the true Guru; and it is by the grace of Guru and one's regular efforts that one realizes the God. In fact every thing happens with the grace of God. A Guru is merely an instrument of God to perform His duty.

God suffers too, caused by the separation of our soul from Him and due to our indifferent attitude to ignore Him. Why we have denied our love to Him? Why should we not suffer for this?

Never Forget God

In both your good and bad times, never forget God. If something happens against your desire or will, do not blame God for it. All the good or bad events, hardships, failures, successes, achievements, diseases, losses and accidents etc. are simply the fruit of our past actions as per the *karmic-law* and have nothing to do with God. When your desires are fulfilled and you are enjoying all kinds of worldly pleasures, even then do not forget God. All the worldly wealth, we are getting and enjoying is coming from God, out of His divine love and mercy upon us. Remember, without His divine mercy we cannot take even our next breathe in this world. We should prove our worthiness of His Divine Love.

God's love is unbiased, eternal, universal and all embracing like a universal loving mother. We do not know that during our past and present lives we might have committed so many sins. Only the intense fire of our deep prayer, repentance and love for God can wipe out our fruits of past misdeeds and God can forgive us for our past mistakes. Since everything in the universe is the manifestation of God Himself, including all living-beings, we must love and appreciate His whole creation too.

Our heart, if pure is the best temple of God. In the depth of silence we can whisper, talk, communicate, and express our feelings & love to God who is sitting in our heart. To convey our feelings to Him and to get His blessings too, no language is needed. The hidden universal silent language of heart does everything.

What is Aum or Om?
What are Anahat Sounds?
What is Laya Yoga?

Om or the *Word* or *Amen* or *Amin* is the first vibratory manifestation of the almighty God Brahman. Before the creation of the universe only God (Brahman) was there in unmanifested form. Om is the first cosmic viberation of God. It is the sound of the whirl of the universal cosmic motor of creation. The cosmic creative motor is working in the universe and Aum is its resulting sound. The sound of Aum is not audible by the human ears. The frequency of Om sound is beyond the audible frequency range. Ordinary sound created by a vibrating object is known as *Ahat* (sound which is produced by striking an object with another and due to the vibration in the object). In all there are *ten* different types of sounds audible by the inner ears during deep meditation known as *Anahat sounds* (sound which have no physical source of viberation). Has any scientist ever do any research work on these ten Anahat sound? Probably no.

Out of ten **Anahat** sounds two or three Anahat sounds are easily audible by every body during the peaceful nights and meditation. But the others are audible only during the deep meditation. If we are awakened suddenly during night, try to listen these *Anahat* sounds immediately. You will listen many of these *Anahat* sounds even if you close your ears. These are the inner sounds of consciousness and not external physical sounds. The technique of meditation through the concentration of our mind on these Anahat sounds is known as **Laya Yoga**. The seekers of God should try it.

Aum sound is all pervading in the universe, but is different from the physical sounds. Any physical sound cannot travel in the vacuum or space, but the Aum sound can. Remember that the Aum sound is subtler than the ether, intelligence, cosmic forces and our thoughts. *Aum created the ether. Ether created the space. The space (Akasha) throughout the universe is filled with ether. The space is not a vacuum. Space created fire, fire created air, air created water and water created earth.*

Om → Ether → Space → Fire → Air → Water → Earth

Our body is made of these five elements i.e. Earth, Water, Air, Fire and Space. Since Aum sound is the subtlest of all these elements, therefore it cannot be detected by any physical scientific instrument and is unheard by our ears. But the yogis can listen *Anahat* sounds during the deep meditation. These *Anahat* sounds are not detectable, as a doctor cannot detect the pain, joy, pleasure and sorrow by any physical instrument. Aum sound develops the intuitive (sixth sense) power of man. There is little intuitive power already in all the men, but it is not so developed that it can be used frequently. But by deep meditation the intuitive power of man get fully developed.

The chanting of *Aum* with human voices is not actually the Aum sound. It is just the imitation of the real cosmic vibratory Aum sound. Chanting of Aum sound helps us in listening the real inner Aum sound. We can know God, if we can utter or repeat the *Aum* sound mentally (*Japa*) during meditation. *Remember Aum is the best name of God.*

Harmony with Nature
And Becoming One with All

All the Scriptures advise man to live in harmony with the Nature. All the creatures including man are made from the five basic elements from the kingdom of God, such as Space, Air, Water, Fire and Earth. All the species are made independent of others and has not been evolved from others as claimed by Charles Darwin. But all the species depend upon each other for their mutual existence. Now the scientists are convinced that Darwin befooled the world for nearly a century and has caused a great harm in the exploration of knowledge of creation of living beings. For a peaceful and happy existence there must be harmony between *all the creation and the Creator too*. But it is a matter of sorrow that this balance has been disturbed due to the follies of human beings.

The planet earth is the sanctuary for the evolution of the human body development and the spiritual involution of the soul (a journey back to God). All the life forms are the expression of God, and are evolving back to God. The first step towards our involution of soul is the realization of oneness with all the living and non-living, feeling of vastness with the universe and lives in harmony with every creation of God with the motto *'live and let live'*.

Can we achieve this Oneness? Yes, we can, by bringing harmony with the Mother Nature in our day-today activities. In the 'Divine Plan of God' by our constant yogic practice, we are blessed with a divine wisdom by expanding our consciousness to include the total creation of God within us. God is the subject for our wisdom. Universal consciousness becomes individual consciousness due to the impact of *'Maya'* and our negative thoughts like jealousy, anger, guilt, greed and ego. We can achieve victory over the five gross elements of creation through yoga, after awakening the Kundalini.

Harmony with
The Five Gross Elements of Creation

The creation from God's five gross elements is in sequence:
God → Om → Ether → Space → Fire → Air → Water → Earth

The Harmony with Earth: The 'Spirit of Earth' is the Mother Earth. It provides the foundation and basis for all life forms. God created Mother Earth for holding us comfortably and for providing food, air, water and all our day-today needs to survive. We should thank Mother Earth for providing all these, before taking our food all the time. We should stop disturbing the natural harmony and creating all kinds of pollutions (air, water, noise, ecological, ethical and others) on earth. This can be achieved, by minimizing our needs to survive, by all of us, and to extract the minimum resources from the earth-crust and it's atmosphere.

The Harmony with Water: The 'Spirit of Water' (vital fluids) on Earth is the most essential element for the evolution of life. Most of the life has evolved in water. The body of the most of the living beings consists of 80% of water element. Water is a purifying element also. It purifies our body also. We should pray the 'sprit of water' to wash and purify our body & our thoughts from the unwanted energies. Pray this spirit to wash our emotional stress, our heart to bring abundance in our lives. Stop wasting and polluting water. Use it carefully for your survival.

The Harmony with Air: The 'Spirit of Air' is associated with our mental aspects like intellect, thoughts and emotions. We should pray the 'Spirit of Air' to purify these. We should be careful and avoid using insulting language to others, avoid reading dirty books with negative thoughts and avoid viewing dirty TV programs and films. Do not pollute the Air. Live in a pollution free air in a green and un-crowded place.

The Harmony with Fire: The 'Spirit of Fire' is the powerful element to melt, burn and transform into their true nature. It burns the negative emotions like: envy, greed, jealousy, anger and hatred etc and to realize the radiant light of God. Pray the 'Spirit of Fire' to purify us by simply constantly looking and gazing at the fire flame.

The Harmony with Space: The 'Spirit of Space (*Ether*)' reminds our vast infinite potential. It is limitless. The whole creation of the universe is suspended in the *Ether* element. Sky is the 'Divine Umbrella' to protect us and created by God. It is always stretched over us to protect us. Concentrate and visualize the vastness of sky with all the Planets, Stars and Galaxies inside, pray to become one with the whole universe and the *Ether*.

Love the whole creation around you. Try to talk with the mountains, rivers, trees, plants, animals, fruits, vegetables, herbs, stars, sun, moon, atoms and molecules and every thing. Everything is alive within the consciousness of God. Try to understand the bond of relationship and interdependence of all the creation with each other. The whole creation is nothing but God Himself. He has materialized Himself from formless to form, under the impact of His '*Maya*'.

Possession of a Human Soul By some other Soul

According to *Bhagwad Geeta* and '*The Tibetan Book of the Dead*' our soul remains in the *bardo* state after our death and till next incarnation. During the *bardo* state it reviews its past lives and decides a suitable model for next birth it deserves. Later at the appropriate time, when the vibrations in the ether are in tune with the requirement of the model of the proposed life, the birth of the soul takes place. It is not necessary that a human soul will take next birth only in the human form. It may be in the form of any other millions of living species. The birth in the next living being is based upon the fruits of past karmas.

Many of us has observed that a human soul is possessed by some other powerful soul. All of a sudden the man begins to behave strangely and utter strange words in a strange voice. After some time the man becomes normal but does not remember any thing of his previous strange behavior. The past memory and knowledge of the man is washed out. But the body of the man remains the same. We are unable to understand such a strange phenomenon. The possessing soul may be the soul of a ghost or a noble man or a deity.

Many times the deities also chose a human soul to convey the divine knowledge or messages or some prophesy to the humanity. Such a possessed human is generally known as a messenger or a prophet. He may not be a divine spiritual man or an aspirant to know God. There have been numerous persons unconcerned to God and randomly chosen, who speak strange divine massage, when possessed by a holy spirit. Such numerous messengers have no right to start a new religion on the basis of their little insignificant massage conveyed to them by a holy-spirit. .

It should be understood clearly that it is not at all a symptom of awakening of the Kundalini or of self-realization of the man. Such a man is neither a saint nor the seeker of God nor a holy man nor he has purified his body to know God. Such a man is absolutely the same like others. He will not get even salvation after his death. But after awakening the Kundalini and piercing the chakras man becomes a super-man with so many miraculous powers (*siddhies*) and it is a door for the salvation of human soul to merge with God.

"God has given us only one mind & one brain. We may devote it to any thing, we like. It's entirely upto us to devote it to either God or to worldly pleasures. God has given us the total freedom to decide & act in this regard. God will neither help nor interfere in this matter."

"Without the acceptance of the existence of God our science is lame and blind. It reduces a man to an insignificant identity as compared to the vastness of the universe. Contrarily, if the science accepts the existence of God, it becomes a beacon of knowledge, then it leads to self-realization of man, after which, the whole universe will become an insignificant drop in the vast ocean of Spirit of man. How wonderful it is?"

*"All know that a drop merges into the ocean but very few know that the ocean also merges into the drop, as '**the action and reaction are equal and opposite**'. We all are the images of God and inside His Dream. Other way God is also within us sitting in our heart. When we watch the wave, we don't see the ocean beneath the waves; but when you watch the whole ocean, we see only one ocean beneath all the innumerable waves. In fact the ocean & the waves are one, only the turbulent Maya (ignorance) has separated both. During the merger of Kundalini with Sahasrara one can realize this truth after becoming one with the ocean of Spirit beneath all the waves of lives."* [1]

! Om Anandam Om!

---

[1] Paragraph from the book "God and Self-realization" (Scientific & Spiritual View) by Sh. Dharam Vir Mangla.

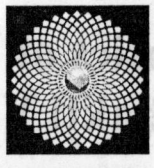

3

The Basics of Kriya
& Bhakti Yoga

Prayer

Yogiraj Sri Mahavatar Babaji
   (Revivalist of the lost Science of Kriya Yoga)

The Basics of Kriya Yoga

Basics of Bhakti Yoga
   (Yoga with Devotion & Worshipping of God)

3
The Basics of Kriya & Bhakti Yoga

Prayer

O Divine Spirit of Creation! What beautiful games you play! Show me the fastest and easiest path of eternal enlightenment. Teach me to dive into vast-cosmic-spaces and the deep-sea-bottoms of silent communion with Thee. Open the petalled centers of our chakras and let our imprisoned soul meet Thee.

O King of all our ambitions! Break the limiting boundary of my consciousness and unite it with Thy Super-Consciousness so that I may become one with all the planets, stars, galaxies and the universe.

Teach me to follow a super-fast path to achieve the ultimate aim in this short span of my life. Without Thy grace it is impossible to wash out all the accumulated fruits of my past actions (karmas) in one life. But nothing is impossible for Thou art. There is no wonder that with Thy grace, I can swim the great dark Ocean of Maya in no time and I will swim forever in Thy enchanting light.

Yogiraj Sri Mahavatar Babaji
(Revivalist of the lost Science of Kriya Yoga)

Sri Mahavatar Baba Ji is an incarnation of Lord *Shiva* in the modern times and he is the great deathless, eternal yogi Guru from India. He lives in the Himalayas above snow line. Babaji is the most revered, miraculous and spiritually advanced Himalayan Yogi. He has earned a great respect among the yogis. He is the guru of Sri Lahari Mahashyia, who was the grand Guru of Sri Paramhansa Yogananda. Sri Mahavtar Babaji came in textual context form first time through '*The Autobiography of a Yogi*' by Sri Paramhansa Yogananda. His age is said to be in **millennium**. Babaji is still a mystery to the world. He has a very attractive look. *He looks like a yogi saint of 25-50 years only. He doesn't eat, doesn't drink anything, doesn't need sleep, doesn't get tired, and doesn't need rest. He appears and disappears at any place at any time as per his will. Whatever he says must happen.*

There is no historical reference to Babaji, because he doesn't appear publicly before the masses and remains away from publicity and media. No body knows actually about his family, time & place of birth and age. He doesn't publicize himself. As he doesn't have any time bound program. It is most difficult to find and meet him, without his grace. He has no ashram, no residence, nor any address and contact number. But he used to materialize and dematerialize many different bodies, out of his body (known as incarnations). Many times he used to disappear at his will for months together from his disciples. Even his close disciples remain without any information about him. But Babaji has assured his devoted disciples that he will appear before them whenever they really *need* him but not when they *want* to meet him. Babaji is in ever communion with Jesus Christ.

Nobody knows about his next program and the place of availability. Without his permission and grace, no body can meet him. None of his actual photograph or picture is available. He has the divine powers to cure anybody and even give life to dead persons.

Once, Mahavatar Babaji has said to His disciples, *"He is deathless. Death has nothing to do with Him. He is the death of the Death. He is the whole universe and the whole universe is inside Him. There is nothing in the universe other then Him. He is present everywhere. He can do whatever He wills. The whole universe is just an expanding bubble ready to burst before Him."*

The technique of Kriya Yoga is one of the greatest contributions of India to World, in the field of spiritual practices. The Kriya Yoga is an ancient spiritual science known to Indian Rishies from the very beginning of evolution of life on earth. It had been lost in dark ages of the vast time-span, but was rediscovered and reestablished by Lord Krishna (5033 yrs ago) and now by Sri Mahavatar Babaji in the 19th century.

In the present world cycle, Babaji has been chosen by God to remain in his physical body for a very long duration of time and to plan & look after, the saints & seers in this delusive world. In modern times the technique of Kriya Yoga was revealed to Sri Lahari Mahashyia[*] in 1861 and many other saints, through the eternal Guru Sri Mahavtar

---

[*] Regarding Sri Lahari Mahashyia, Adi Shankaracharaya, Heda Khan Babaji and Amar Jyoti Babaji read the book 'God & Self-Realization' (Scientific & Spiritual View) by Dharam Vir Mangla.

Babaji. *Sri Lahari Mahashyia* **was further authorized by Babaji to transfer it, to the whole world (including women), through his authorized disciples.** Kriya Yoga discipline is strict, but Babaji relaxed it on the request of Sri Lahari Mahashyia. Babaji relented and advised Lahari Mahashyia to freely initiate all those who seek spiritual enlightenment. Householders were allowed for initiation in Kriya Yoga, but there is requirement of his deservingness. A disciple takes a new birth after initiation; just as a seed takes new birth after sprouting.

Babaji told Sri Lahari Mahashyia, "Kriya Yoga is a revival of the same lost science that Krishna gave millennium ago to Arjuna; and that was later known to Maharishi Patanjali, Jesus Christ, Saint John, St. Paul, Sri Heda Khan Babaji, Sri Amar Jyoti Babaji, Shiv Goraksha Babaji and Yogiraj Gurunath." It is said that Babaji also initiated the seers like Adi-Shankaracharaya and Kabir in Kriya yoga. There are so many other saints unknown to the world, who were also directly initiated by Babaji in *Kriya Yoga*.

Maharishi Patanjali is the great exponent and ancient author of yoga. He has predominantly prescribed Kriya yoga in his aphorisms. Now there are so-many ashrams, which provide this technique to their disciples. Lord Krishna in Srimad Bhagwad Geeta, has also mentioned about the path of Kriya Yoga at many places:

The same Lord Krishna in his previous incarnation communicated this eternal knowledge of yoga to an ancient Rishi *Vivasvat*. He gave it further to Manu, the great legislator. Manu gave it further to the king *Ikshwaku*. *Ikshwaku* further passed on this knowledge to *Harshchandra*, *Rama* and several *Rishies*. But due the impact of *Maya*, its secrecy and long span of time, it gradually disappeared became inaccessible to the ordinary seekers of God.

> The Sloka IV: 29 means: "The aspirants who are interested to practice the control of breath (pranayama) to remain in trance achieve, by offering the movement of the outgoing breath into the incoming breath, and the incoming breath into the outgoing breath. The aspirant try to neutralizes his both the incoming and outgoing breaths. He releases extra prana to the body and brings the life force under his control."

> Another Sloka means: "An aspirant who seeks his ultimate eternal goal of making him free from all bondages, if he withdraws the life force from his senses (the external world), by fixing his gaze at the mid point of the eyes brows (Aggyia chakra), by neutralizing the currents of *prana* & *apana* within the nostrils (Ida & Pingla) and lungs; and to control his sensory mind and intellect; and to banish his desires, fear, and anger."

The Basics of Kriya Yoga

Yoga is the technique of verification and realization of a true religion. The true religion of God is not simply a collection of do's and don'ts dictated by the Head/ Founder of religions. It must be verifiable through Yoga. Kriya yoga is such and is one of the powerful and fastest paths of divine union attained through the uplift of limited human consciousness to cosmic consciousness. It is a specialized scientific technique of breathing with concentration on chakras along with meditation. It is different from forcibly holding, retaining and exhaling breath in lungs, unnaturally and unscientifically during the practice of pranayama, taught by most of the asana teachers. The practice of pranayama is generally uncomfortable and unpleasant, while the practice of Kriya gives joy, bliss, peace, happiness and a soothing sensation in the spine.

As per some restrictions of the Scriptures, Kriya Yoga technique is not for everyone, but only for the deserving one. Only those aspirants, who are seriously interested in seeking God, should practice the Kriya technique. The details of this technique may be provided through e-mail to the authorized members* of GRF, if they qualify the GRF e-Spiritual Tests, especially designed for this purpose.

The *'Kriya'* is a Sanskrit word. *'Kri'* means to do, to perform or to act & react. 'Yoga' means union of soul with God. Thus Kriya Yoga means the union of soul with God through certain actions or practices by the aspirant.

Kriya Yoga is a specialized breathing technique mixed with concentration and meditation, by the aspirants. It is generally taught only to the deserving & eligible disciples through the authorized Gurus at the time of their initiation (*Diksha*). Because of certain ancient yogic injunctions, general public who is unconcerned with God is not entitled to practice this technique. The yogis who practice Yam-Niyama, Asanas, Pranayama and Meditation regularly are entitled to get *Diksha* in Kriya Yoga and they are known as *Kriyaban*.

As per Maharishi Patanjali, there are three essential components of Kriya yoga. *"Tapasya, Swadhyay & Ishwarpranidhan*. These three are not independent, but

---

* See the instructions to become the authorized member of God-Realization Foundation (GRF) at pages 231-2.

interdependent on each other. Here Tapasya does not mean to go to forest, leave the home & family, and escape from worldly responsibilities. Kriya yoga is very well for the householders and office goers. Sri Lahari Mahashyia himself was also a householder. *Swadhyay* means self-study of Scriptures like Vedas, Geeta, Upanishads and Brahma-sutras etc. *Ishwarpranidhan* means one should always love and think of God in each of his breath".

So many ancient yogis of India discovered the spiritual secret: "Self-realization and cosmic super-consciousness are intimately linked and connected with the mastery over the breathing known as pranayama". By this specialized technique of meditation, concentration and breathing, the aspirants are able to de-carbonized, over-oxygenized and over-charged their blood with *pranic energy*. *Prana* doesn't mean air or oxygen in air or breathing as generally misunderstood, but it is the omnipresent universal life-energy.

Due to this life-energy, there is an evolution of life in all the living species. The physical bodies and brains are changing and the faculties of mind are developing. The rate normal evolution of this change is very slow. But this slow evolution of man can be tremendously increased by the Kriya-Yoga technique.

The consciousness of an ordinary man identifies itself with his senses, physical body and outer world. By regular practice of Kriya yoga the consciousness is transformed inside the spine and brain. Human consciousness is first transmuted into super-consciousness and ultimately into cosmic-consciousness of God. After that a yogi will realize and understand that not only within his inner-self, the whole outer restless material world and universe is also the manifestation of same God. God is both within and without us.

The hidden astral body of the human beings is equipped with the six inner chakras in spine, twelve constellations and the inner 'third eye' also known as 'spiritual eye'. All these are interrelated with the outer external twelve zodiacal signs and the physical sun in the sky. All these affect and control the events of our life and destiny. Planets also affect our future evolution.

The evolution of one cycle takes twelve years in a natural way. But the evolution by one Kriya practice is equivalent of one-solar-year natural evolution. Fourteen Kriya practice in one sitting are equivalent to twelve years of natural evolution of man. In this way a Kriya yogi achieves a million years of natural evolution, just in three years of Kriya practice. It is strange.

There is nothing like absolute-time. Time is also relative as per Theory of Relativity. If one of the twins travels out into space with a speed closer to speed of light and return after 10 yrs of his space journey, he will find that his twin on earth has become 50 or more yrs older than him. The time elapsed for the twins will be quite different. In the same way this time limitation of slow human evolution is overcome by the practice of Kriya by the aspirants.

Kriya technique is a shortcut and a faster journey by a concord plane as compared to other techniques, which are like the slow journey on foot. In this way a Kriya yogi achieves freedom from bondages within his lifetime instead of waiting for millions of years of natural living in human form.

All the fruits of our past actions of this life and the previous lives are stored in our Sushumana nadi, just like a huge data is hiddenly stored in a computer Hard-Disk. In this life we take our birth and rewards according to the fruits of our past actions *(karmas)*. Unless we erase or delete all the accumulated fruits of past actions by enjoying or suffering, we cannot enter the kingdom of God. The Kriya practice erases or wipes out our fruits of past actions in Sushumana Nadi as the files are deleted in computer Hard-Disk. So a Kriya yogi is able to, neutralize the fruits of millions of years of past karmas in the short span of his life and achieves enlightenment at the earliest.

The body of an ordinary man is like a sixty watts electric bulb and his body is not able to sustain thousands of watts of energy generated by the excessive Kriya practice. Due to the Kriya practice the physical body of an aspirant is gradually transformed into astral body, which is able to tolerate the extra high energy generated during Kriya. So an aspirant should begin with fourteen Kriyas initially and gradually increase it to 24 or 48 with the permission of his experienced Guru.

Through a specialized breathing (pranayama) meditation Kriya technique, the blood is decarbonized and over-charged with oxygen. The extra atoms of oxygen in blood are transmuted into life-current to rejuvenate the brain and the subtle chakras in Sushumana. By Kriya technique an aspirant is able to reduce and prevent the decay of tissue cells, by stopping the accumulation of de-oxygenated blood in his veins. Yogi achieves the state of suspended animation. Many advanced aspirants are able to transmute these cells into life-energy.

The Basics of Kriya & Bhakti Yoga

Through regular Kriya practice a yogi gets the control & mastery over the prana energy. A Kriya yogi is able to disconnect his mind from his five senses and his body organs. He is able to tune his consciousness to the six higher centers of perceptions in the spine. A Kriya yogi withdraws the life energy from his body and meditates on chakras in the spine. It produces perfect sensory nerves relaxation.

A Kriya Yogi tries to energize his spine forcefully by up and down flow of the life energy. Side by side the Kriya yogi tries to withdraw the life energy from his five sense organs, brain and nerves. He tries to store the life energy into his chakras through his will and consciousness. The Kriya technique shifts our attention from the gross sense perceptions to subtle inner perceptions in the mind and nadis. This expands our limited consciousness to super consciousness.

It has been found by the biological scientists that the species, which have a short span of life, are generally restless. They take so many breaths in a minute e.g. monkeys, bees and mosquitoes etc. But on the other side the species with long lives like elephants, tortoise and snakes are peaceful and takes only a few breaths in a minute. Due to the restless mind like a monkey, the life of a man reduced but a peaceful mind with deep breath makes the life of man longer. The Kriya meditation makes the mind of yogi peaceful and calm.

A Kriyaban is able to convert his breath into mind stuff. Then he is further gets the ability to materialize and dematerialize his body cells at his sweet will. Such a yogi gets the power (Sidhhi) to transport, appear and disappear at any place and even after his death. He becomes beyond the relativity of time and space of Einstein.

A huge amount of the life force is generally consumed or wasted in digestion, in pumping of blood by the heart to all the organs of the physical body. By the method of controlling the ceaseless demand of the breath in Kriya practice, the heart and digestion are slowed down and heart is made free from pumping the blood continuously. Life currents are withdrawn from the senses and nerves. This saved a huge amount of life energy by calming the heart, digestion and senses. A Kriya yogi uses this saved life-energy for doing still higher activities like awakening, activating and piercing the chakras by the Kundalini. Kriya practice purifies our body and makes it a divine temple perfectly fit to receive God.

The Cosmic energy of God is the cause of creation of every thing in the universe. It also supplies the life energy secretly to our body to sustain it. Till now the humanity is ignorant of the link between the physical energies, life energy and cosmic energy. Cosmic energy of God is finer than life energy and life energy is finer than all the physical energies and electromagnetic waves existing in nature. All our consciousness, sub-consciousness, unconsciousness and super-consciousness are the manifestation of one cosmic consciousness of God.

Our tiny soul is a microscopic image of the Supreme macroscopic Soul of Brahman, just as a drop of water is the microscopic part of the great ocean. The Supreme-soul first manifests vibrations of super-consciousness, which further vibrates into life energy and it further vibrates into gross-body* of man. How all these vibrations affect each other is a mystery to be understood. This ignorance leads us to presume that mind and matter are quite different. In fact matter is the creation of our own mind. It is most interesting to note that whatever is in the macrocosm is in the microcosm also. All the microcosms are connected with the one whole macrocosm. None has any separate identity excusive of the total universe.

A Kriya yogi must study regularly the sacred scriptures and holy books sent to humanity directly from God. He should not adulterate or pollute his mind by reading the literature of non-believers of 'God & soul' written by those who could not realize God. There are so many who tried to know God but failed in their mission to realize due to their past karmas and then declared that God does not exist due their ignorance. Ignorance can only be destroyed by knowledge of God. If someone fails to realize God is not a proof of non-existence of God.

The universe, matter and our body exist till our mind exists. In our awakening state, mind exists and hence the universe exists around us. During the sleep state our mind is tuned to different frequency of vibrations and then the universe does not exist for us? So it is clear that the matter around us has no real existence as it appears to us. Matter is simply the vibration of life energy as created by the vibrations of consciousness by our mind. If one can control these vibrations, one can fix his mind upon God and is able to materialize and dematerialize his physical body. The control of life energy during Kriya produces a super-conscious state of deep silence. The Kriya yoga technique helps us to realize all these.

---

* Read Chapter Miscellaneous Information

Bhakti Yoga
(The Yoga with Devotion & Worshipping of God)

In Bhakti (devotion) Yoga an aspirant worship either the trinity Brahma, Vishnu and Mahesha or trinity of Goddess Saraswati, Maha-Laxmi and Durga or different Avataras of God like Lord Rama, Lord Krishna, Hanuman, Ganesha & others. Some of the aspirants also worship the great saints, deity-gods etc.

There are two kinds of worshiping known as *Sugun & Nirgun*. The worshiping & meditation on the manifested God and Avataras is known as *Sugun Bhakti*. In Sugun Bhakti there is a duality. God and soul are presumed to be different. God is every thing and the soul is tiny part of it. God is like the Ocean and the soul is just a drop or a wave in the ocean. The devotee tries to lose his identity after merging in the manifested God. God may be presumed in the human manifested form like an Avatara in human form. In Bhakti God plays a divine romance with his disciples. The devotee also completely surrenders to his Lord and becomes like a child at the mercy of Lord.

The worshiping and meditation on the unmanifested God (Brahman) is known as *Nirgun Bhakti*. Brahman is devoid of all the attributes. Nirgun Bhakti is considered as higher form of worshiping God. It is more suitable for the educated intellectuals, who have strong will power and a deep understanding of the concept of God. Ultimately, Nirgun Bhakti becomes the same as *Jnana* (knowledge) Yoga.

Deep devotion is acquired and cultivated through *Bhajans, dancing* and *Satsanga* with saints and a thorough understanding of the concept of God through good spiritual books. As per the scriptures, there are nine methods of developing a strong devotion (*Bhakti*) to God by a devotee. Satsanga with saints, japa of mantras, prayer, meditation, spiritual studies, singing and listening spiritual songs, serving the saints, charity, spiritual tours, etc., will develop devotion for God.

The nine methods of developing devotion (*Bhakti*) are:

Sravana:	Listening the Leelas of Avataras & Shastras
Smarana:	Remembering God always in each breath
Kirtan:	A group singing in the praise of God
Vandana:	Offering prayers and whispering with God
Archana:	Offerings to God
Pada-Sevana:	Attendance
Sakhya:	Friendship with God
Dasya:	Service of God
Atma-Nivedana:	Self-surrender to God and Guru

Some useful measures in the development of devotion are:

Discrimination, strong desire to know God, detachment from worldly things, good to other, good wishes for all, no enmity with any body, truthfulness, integrity, compassion, non-violence and charity to poor.

Meera Bai, Soor Das, Guru Nanak Das, Nam Dev, Ram Das, Tulsi Das and others are the good examples of *Bhaktas* to whom God was revealed. Generally, the great Bhaktas come to the world with their great asset of spiritual *Samskaras*. They had worshipped God in their previous births with sincere devotion. Through devotional prayer, japa, kirtan, service to humanity, charity, fasting, meditation and Samadhi, a devotional yogi should uplift his consciousness to universal consciousness and acquire the highest knowledge of supreme Brahman. In the advanced stage of meditation, the meditator (worshipper) & the object of meditation (the worshipped) become one. Then there will be no difference in the ego 'I' and God and the meditator will enter into samadhi.

A devotee when meditates on the presiding deity, imagines the particular form of god at each chakra. The yogi also gets various subtle visions and observes different forms of God.

"If you could feel once even a spark of divine love, so great would be your joy & bliss...overpowering you ...that you will hanker after Him for the rest of your life. That is why the name of God is Hari (who deprives you of every attachment)."

"The greatest romance one can have is the romance with God, who is the Supreme-Lover and our souls are His beloved. During deep meditation, when our soul meets the greatest Lover of the universe, then the eternal divine romance begins. It is different from sex pleasure which is an animal instinct"

!Om Peace, Peace, Peace!

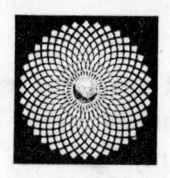

4

The Life-Force, Nadis & Chakras

Prayer
Know Your Spinal Column
Body Cells Need Regular Recharging
What are the *Nadis*?
   1. *Ida* 2. *Pingla* 3. *Sushumana*
Cross-section of Sushumana Nadi
The Symptoms of Sushumana Nadi Activation
Our Body has been Given an Ego 'I'
Five Types of *Pranas* and *Sub-Pranas* in body
What happens to *Prana* After Death?
Medulla Oblongata and Seven Chakras
Reception & Distribution of *Pranas*
Sahasrar (the Reservoir of Life Energy)
Picture of Position of *Nadis & Chakras* in Astral Body

Chakras: Aggyia Chakra, Vishuddha Chakra, Anahat Chakra, Manipur Chakra, Swadhisthan Chakra, Muladhara Chakra.

Prayer

O Spirit Divine, Come Thou in my temple of silence. Thou art just behind the curtain of *Maya*. Thou art my Creator, my Guru, my Teacher, my Soul, my Friend and my Love. Thou art the saint of all religions. Thou saints are Thy incarnation doing Thy work. I bow them all.

Divine Mother! Thou all the laws of science are miraculous, but Thou saints are more miraculous. The each phenomenon of Thy wonderful universe is also miraculous. But my little mind is unable to understand fully, Thy miraculous creation and their mysteries unless Thou help me to understand, through Thy infinite vision.

Thy saints know Thy reality and are beyond Thy *Maya*. Thou hast revealed them Thou secret of wonderful creation. Thou art the Creator of all the laws of nature, science and the universe. Nothing is beyond Thy omnipresent omnipower and nothing is impossible for Thee.

4
The Life-Force, Nadis & Chakras

Know your Spinal Column

The spinal column is the most important organ of physical body, to understand the *Chakras, Nadis* and subtle things in the astral body. All the chakras are connected with it. All the nadis including the main nadis *Id, Pingla* and *Sushumana* are also connected with it. Most of the asanas and the centers of concentration and meditation are situated inside it.

Spinal column is the axis, which supports most of the body structure is linked with most of the body organs. It consists of 33 bones known as vertebras. Vertebras are joined together with nerves and discs arranged in a vertical line. Spine is mainly divided into five regions starting from top to bottom as shown in the diagram: Cervical (7[1]), Thoracic (12), Lumber (5), Sacral (5), Coccygeal (4).

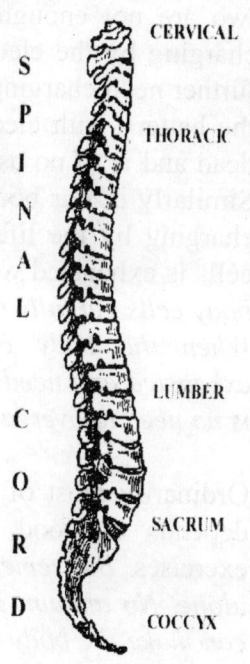

The spine is symbolized as the tree of consciousness, through which flows the sap of life. The spinal cord is the trunk; the cranial nerves are the roots.

---
[1] Number of vertebras

Our Body Cells are like Battery Cells and Need Re-charging

A living body cell is just like a battery cell. It consist of hardware i.e. a physical container and a few chemicals inside it. The chemicals and fluids are supplied to the living cells by the food we take in. For a battery cell, these two are not enough. As a battery cell further needs the charging by the electrical energy, similarly the body cells further need charging by the life energy just like energizing the battery with electricity. Without charging, a battery is dead and is of no use. A dead battery cannot do any work. Similarly in our body, living cells also need energizing or charging by the life energy. When the life energy of the cells is exhausted we are tired. *Always remember when the body cells get fully charged body becomes fresh and active. When the body cells are discharged, body is tired, exhausted and need to go to sleep to re-charge it, but there is no need to overeat for re-charging.*

Ordinarily most of the people think that our body simply depends on food, water, air, heat and some physical exercises. *But remember our body is sustained not by food alone. No amount of food given to a dead body of a man can make the body alive, not even a single body organ will function, since the four out of five life forces are missing in the dead body.*

What are the *Nadis*?

The nadis are in the astral body made up of astral subtle matter that carries the psychic currents. The *pranic* currents (vital force) flow through these nadis. Since the nadis are not made up of any physical matter and are not the ordinary physical nerves, the doctors are not able to detect these in the physical body. Overall there are 72,000 to 3,50,000 nadis and sub-nadis in the astral body of man. Since the nadis play a vital role in the awakening of the Kundalini, therefore aspirants should first purify the nadis. Nadi has a tubular structure consisting of three layers, one over the other. The outer layer is called *nadi*, the middle one is called *Damini* and the innermost central layer is called *Sira*.

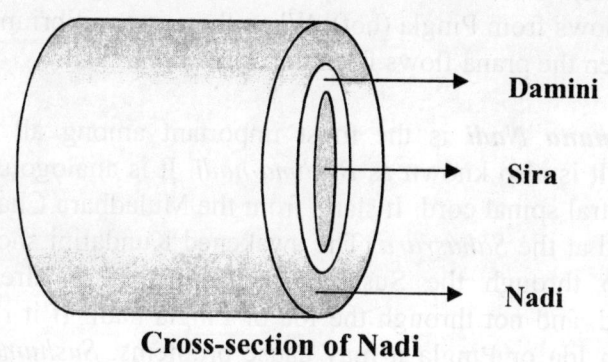

Cross-section of Nadi

There are fourteen main nadis. But the following three are the most important nadis:

    1. Ida   2. Pingla   3. Sushumana

Ida & Pingla Nadis are the nadis, which carry the subtle prana. The Ida (moon) starts from the right testicle and the Pingla (sun) starts from the left testicle. Both meet the Sushumana nadi at the *Muladhara Chakra* and make a knot there. These nadis again meet at *Anahat* and *Aggyia* Chakra. Ida (cool) flows through the left nostril and the Pingla (hot) flows from the right nostril.

Ida is also known as moon-nadi as it is cool in nature. It controls the high blood pressure and overflow of bile juice. Pingla is also known as sun-nadi as it is hot in nature. It maintains the blood pressure and activates the digestive system.

In a healthy man both Ida & Pingla nadis work together in harmony with each other for maintaining the body temperature, odour and blood pressure etc. Ida & Pingla Nadis carry the prana and apana.

When we breathe from the left nostril, prana flows through Ida (cool). But when we breathe from the right nostril, prana flows from Pingla (hot). When there is equilibrium in both then the prana flows from the *Sushumana* Nadi.

Sushumana Nadi is the most important among all the Nadis. It is also known as *Brahma nadi*. It is analogous to the central spinal cord. It starts from the Muladhara Chakra and end at the *Sahasrara*. The awakened Kundalini should rise up through the Sushumana nadi, if it is already purified, and not through the Ida or Pingla nadi. If it rises through Ida or Pingla it may cause problems. *Sushumana* has the equilibrium with both *Ida & Pingla*. The innermost central core of Sushumana is known as *Brahman Nadi*.

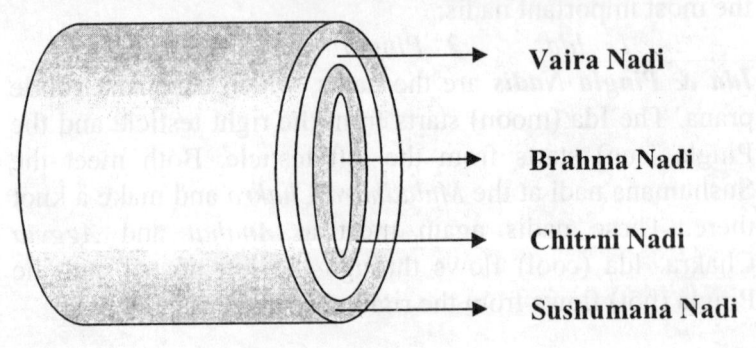

Vaira Nadi
Brahma Nadi
Chitrni Nadi
Sushumana Nadi

Cross-section of Sushumana Nadi

All the physical and cosmic vibrations in the entire universe are echoed in our subtle etheric body. The subtle body further affects our physical body, which is analogous to etheric body. The impact of vibrations that flow around our body affect the karmic deeds (fruits of past karmas) stored in Brahman Nadi. These further affect the prana flowing in the nadis and chakras. All our karmic deeds are stored in the central *Sushumana* Nadi known as Brahma nadi in the form of miniature astral body known as *Suksham-Sharira* (the miniature body).

The Symptoms of Sushumana Nadi Activation

When the Sushumana Nadi of an aspirant is activated and purified the following symptoms occurs:
- The mind of the person is automatically detached from the enchanting worldly things.
- There is a visible glow on the face of the person.
- An attractive aura is developed around his body.
- The person gets a victory over most of his diseases.
- The aspirant becomes more spiritual and peaceful.

Our Body has also been given an Ego 'I' or *Ahankar*

All mighty God has assigned each soul with a physical living body and by His delusive power associated a separate ego known as 'I' or *Ahankar*. God has separated each soul from Himself due to His delusive power of *Maya*. *Maya* separates the creation from the Creator by creating ignorance. Our soul is associated with an ego 'I'. The ego 'I' is not our physical body. Any thing, which is mine, can never be 'I'. I am always different from my things, which are mine. All the things like my shirt, my car, my ears, my nose, my tongue, my hands, my legs, my brain, my mind, my intelligence are due to *Maya*. None of these is my real 'I'.

No part of my physical body is 'I'. Our ego 'I' is surrounded by the ignorance due to *Maya* created by Almighty God to separate us for Him. Only by our continuous efforts of yoga, love & devotion and the grace of God, we can remove this ignorance of duality ('I' & God are different) and our separation from God. We must remember that *Maya separates us form God, but love and devotion unites us with God.*

When Kundalini is awakened then during **samadhi** ignorance is removed, the ego 'I' is dissolved in the ocean of cosmic waves of God. The yogi realizes that there is no difference between his ego 'I' and the Almighty God. When the ego 'I' merges in God soul becomes one with God (*Advaita* Philosophy), then the yogi realizes the absolute state of *Brahman* i.e. *Sat, Chit* and *Ananda*. During this state we experience and realize the great powers of God i.e. omnipresence, omnipotence, omniscience etc. We realize that the whole universe is my physical body. We will experience that I am present everywhere and all living beings are inside me. Further there is nothing other then me in the universe. We will come to know each and every thing about the whole universe.

Remember it is only in this state of consciousness that we can really realize the great statements of Vedas like: "You and 'I' are One" or *"Aham Brahmasmi"* or *"So-Ham"* or "Shiv-o-ham" or *"Tatvamasi"*. *Remember without the victory over the ego 'I', one can't realize the truth of above great statements of Vedas.*

Five Types of Sub-Pranas are Working in our Living Body

Generally we know that the food, sunrays, air, fluids & juices etc. sustain a living body. But the most important apart from these is *the vital infinite intelligent life force (prana)*. Prana is the sum total of all energy that is manifested in the universe. It is a vital force. Prana does not mean breath or air. But by the control of breath one can control the prana. The control of prana also controls the mind.

The prana is related to mind; through mind to the will; through will to the individual soul and through soul to the God. Prana has to do so many functions in the universe including our body, mind and sprit.

There are two kinds of *'prana'*:

(1) **Main Life Force** (*Main-prana*): It is the cosmic vibratory energy. It is present throughout the universe even inside the living cells, atoms, molecules and elementary particles etc. It structures, organizes and sustains every thing in the livings, non-livings and inert matter throughout the universe.

(2) **The Specific Life Forces** (sub-*pranas*): It prevails and sustains our physical body. These are the sum total of all latent forces which are hidden in men and which lie everywhere around us. These are of five types of life currents depending on their functions in our body. The following are the five *sub-pranas*:
   ➢ *Prana* current controls crystallization and chest perspiration.
   ➢ *Vyana* current helps circulation of blood in whole body.

> *Samana* current helps assimilation, induces hunger & thrust.
> *Udana* current helps metabolism, separates the physical body from the astral body.
> *Apana* current helps elimination of urine, sweating and faeces etc.

All the above five *sub-pranas* have further five, *sub-sub-pranas*.

What Happens to *Pranas* after Death?

Charak Rishi has said: *"All those born shall die and will born again, till he washouts the fruits of his karmic deeds".*

At the time of death, the moment the soul leaves our body; four out of five sub-*pranas* leave the dead body. Only the *Udana sub-prana* remains in the body to destroy the dead body into further five elements: earth, water, air, fire and space from which it is made up of. Nothing can perish automatically without this prana. The dead organic materials are destroyed due to this prana, but the plastics do not destroy easily due to its absence. This is a great ecological problem of the world. Our earth would have been a hell or a big storage of dead bodies in the absence of this important *Udana sub-prana*. Remember that *the injuries or diseases of a dead body can never be repaired or cured by any medicine given after the death due to the absence of other four sub-pranas.*

Even the injuries of a living body are not repaired by any medicine however costly it is. It is the life force inside the living body, which repairs the injuries of the living body or cures the body. The medicines simply help and protect the body from the infection caused due to external or internal bacterias. The medicines may also cure the deficiency diseases. Most of the medicines and the treatment simply help in activating the life force in the sick part of the body. The body is repaired and cured by the life force having infinite intelligence and not by the medicine and the treatments given to the body.

In physiotherapy treatment life-force is activated in the required organ of the body. No physiotherapy can help in a dead body where four of the life forces (sub-*pranas*) are missing. *Remember it is the infinite intelligent life force, which knows what to do and how to cure a diseased body and not the inert blind medicine, which is void of any intelligence.*

It is now clear to us why we are tired during the awakening state, even if we take enough food and do not work throughout the day? Further why we become fresh and energetic again, in the morning after a peaceful sleep during night, without taking any food? **It seems to be a paradox. But what is our tiredness exactly?** Science needs to do further research work to understand it deeply.

To understand the above paradox, we have to understand first, how our body is receiving the life force and how it is stored, consumed or spend by the body? From where the life force is coming? Which organ of our body receives the life force? How & who distributes this life force in different parts of our body as per its requirement?

Medulla Oblongata & The Seven *Chakras* in the Body

The most important part of our body **is the medulla oblongata**. It is also known as **'the mouth of God'** or **'the seat of soul'** (*Atam-singhasan*). It is situated at the top end of our spinal cord, at the centre of cerebrum. For safety a

seat of soul' (*Atam-singhasan*). It is situated at the top end of our spinal cord, at the centre of cerebrum. For safety a fluid surrounds it. It is the centre of all the centers of life, in the brain and spine. Medulla oblongata is like the radio or TV antenna or the receiver of the life force from the cosmos. The other centers of the body are not the receiver but the storehouse & distributor of the life force, which has been received by medulla oblongata.

The chakras are the vortex of psychic energy. These can be visualized as a circular movement of energy at a particular rate of vibration. Anatomically, chakras are like the junctions of the nerves/ nadis where these meet. There are six important centers of distribution of life energy inside our Astral or Ethereal Body, but not in the physical body. The doctors cannot find these centers, inside the physical body, as these centers are not the physical material things. The advance yogis can experience these centers of life forces, during deep meditation state. These are known as *Chakras*. Chakras are like the poles of electricity through which electrical wires (nadis) run across to supply power at different centers. Through nadis the vital energy flows. There are six *chakras* corresponding to life-force centers inside our brain and spine. But according to some Sahasrara is not a Chakra. Chakras are as follows:

Physical Body Organ	Corresp. *Chakra*	Beej Mantra of Chakra
1. Coccygeal	*Muladhar*	*LAM*
2. Lumber	*Swadhisthan*	*VAM*
3. Dorsal	*Manipur*	*RAM*
4. Heart	*Anahat*	*YAM*
5. Cervical	*Vishuddha*	*HAM*
6. Fore Head	*Aggyia*	*OM*
7. Top of Brain	*Sahasrar*	

Reception & Distribution of Life-Energy (*Prana*)

Sahasrar: It is not a chakra. But many call it the 7th chakra. It is the most important thousand-patelled lotus situated at the top of the brain. It is known as the "Hole of Brahman" and the dwelling house of the human soul. It is like the *reservoir or the storage of the cosmic life force* for the body. It is like the UPS / inverter for the power supply of the computer. It is experienced as the thousand-patelled lotus at the top of the brain to the yogis. From this life force is released or supplied to the body whenever it is required urgently in case of emergency.

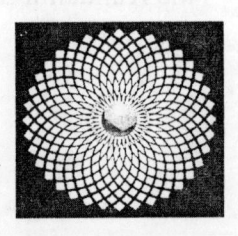

At the time of death, if yogi concentrates at the Sahasrara, his soul pierces through it, it bursts and open. The soul of the yogi merges with Brahman and the yogi become immortal forever.

Some times a person with a heavy blow or injury in the head may see the thousands of stars of light, due to the forceful displacement of this stored energy in *Sahasrar*. At the time of death, the soul of some of the advanced yogis leave out of their physical body through the *Sahasrar* by breaking the top of their head. The soul of such a yogi is merged with God after leaving the body.

Our brain and mind are like *TV tuner*, which tunes our mind to different cosmic wavelengths or states of consciousness like awakening, dream sleep, deep sleep & meditation etc. But the medulla oblongata is like a *TV antenna,* a receiver of the cosmic life currents. After receiving the life energy vibrations, these are reflected at the *Aggyia Chakra* situated in our forehead. Sahasrara is the seat of cosmic awareness and is the terminal point of the Kundalini Shakti.

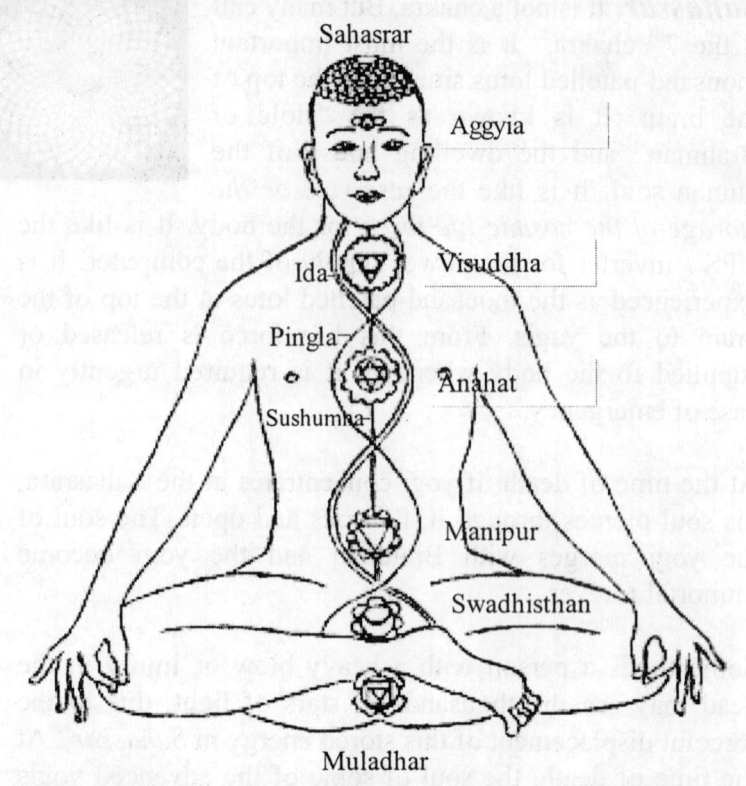

The position of Ida, Pingla, Sushumana Nadis & Seven Chakras in the Spinal Cord of human body

As per Swami Satyananda Saraswati's book 'Kundalini Tantra':
"The serpent power is considered to arise from the unconscious state in *Muladhara*. The unconscious awareness of man then has to pass through different phases and becomes one with the cosmic awareness of man then has to pass through different phases and becomes one with

the cosmic awareness in the highest realm of existence. Lord Shiva is seated as the Supreme awareness, the super consciousness or transcendental body at the crown of the head inside the Sahasrara. In the Vedas, as well as in the Tantras, this supreme seat is called *Hiranyagarbha*, the womb of consciousness. It corresponds to the pituitary master gland situated within the brain. For a Kundalini Yogi, the supreme consciousness represents the highest possible manifestation of physical matter in the body. This psychic, supersensory or transcendental power in man is the ultimate point of human evolution."

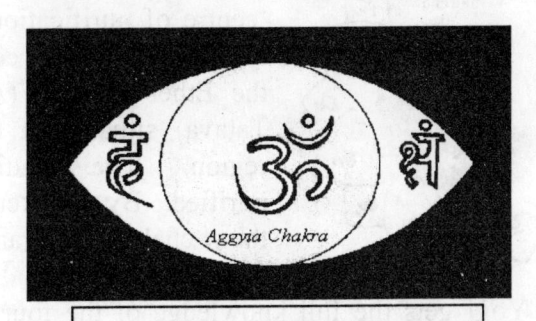

Aggyia Chakra (Aum)

The next 6th *Aggyia chakra* situated at our forehead is also called *'centre of command'*, *'the Eye of Shiva'* or *'The Third Eye'*. There are only two petals of the lotus in this chakra. It converts the main *prana* into five types of sub-*pranas*, reflect and distribute the sub-*pranas* to different parts of the body organs through other *Chakras* as per their requirement. *Aggyia chakra* is like the *power supply* part of the personal computer, which converts the 240V main current into other currents at different voltages as per the requirement of the computer parts. It is related to pineal gland and takes care of all the functions of the body.

The aspirants who concentrate at this Chakra with the Anahat sound of *Om* are able to destroy all the fruits of the actions (*karmas*) of his past lives. Yogi acquires all the 8 major and 32 minor siddhies at this Chakra. The yogi becomes a liberated soul in his lifetime. He gets the *Moksha & the liberation of soul (Jivan-Mukti)*. The ego 'I' still exist at Aggyia chakra.

Vishuddha Chakra
Beej Mantra 'HAM'

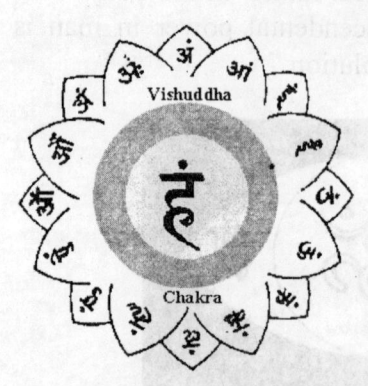

The 5th Chakra is known, as ***Vishuddha Chakra***. It is the 'centre of purification'. It is also known as the centre of the Ether element (Akasha-Tatava) situated at cervical region. The nadis are purified. By awakening of this chakra aspirant gets freedom from 'worldly desires'. Yogi gets the full knowledge of the four Vedas. The past, present and future become known by meditating at this Chakra. It takes care of thyroid gland, upper palate and epiglottis etc.

Anahat Chakra
Beej Mantra 'YAM'

The 4th Chakra is known as ***Anahat Chakra***. It is located at the level of heart (cardiac plexus). It is associated with love and compassion. With the awakening of this chakra one can hear with the inner ear the ten *Anahat* sounds including Om. When the Kundalini pierces this chakra the aspirant gets control over his heart.

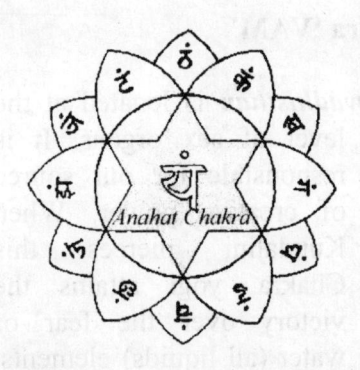

The Anahat Sound, Word, *Shabda or Pranava* (Om) is heard at this Chakra. The yogi gets the control over the air (all gaseous) elements at this Chakra. Yogi gets cosmic love and all other divine pure qualities. It takes care of heart, the lungs and the diaphragm etc. in the body. The yogi gets his control over his next birth. He can choose his parents; take birth in the form of his liking (man or any other living being), at the right time and place of his sweet will. Its Beej Mantra is YAM.

Manipur Chakra
Beej Mantra 'RAM'

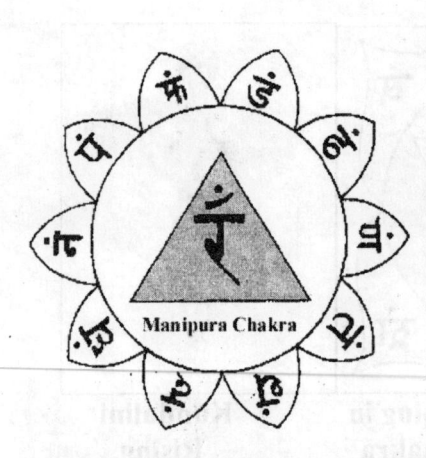

The 3rd Chakra known as *Manipur* is located in the abdominal area. When yogi concentrates at this Chakra, he achieves *Patala Siddhi*. *He becomes free from all diseases and acquires the hidden treasures* below the earth. It looks after the digestive, assimilative and temperature controlling system of the body. Its Beej Mantra is RAM.

Beej mantra 'VAM'

The 2nd Chakra known as *Swadhisthan* is located at the level of sex organs. It is responsible for our source of creative power. When Kundalini pierces this Chakra, yogi attains the victory over the fear of water (all liquids) elements. Yogi gets the intuitional knowledge, mystic psychic powers and a perfect control over his five senses. Yogi gets the complete control over his sex, anger, greed, attachments and proud etc. He gets the victory over his death. Its Beej Mantra is VAM.

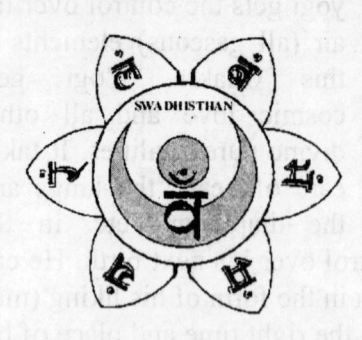

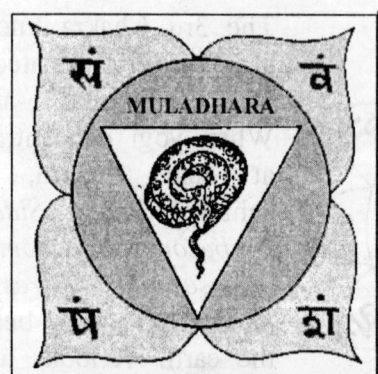

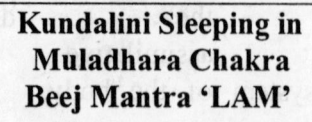

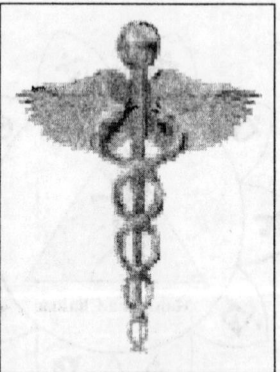

Kundalini Sleeping in Muladhara Chakra Beej Mantra 'LAM'

Kundalini Rising

The 1st Chakra is known as *Muladhara*. It is situated at the lowest point of the spine. It is the seat of the dormant *Kundalini Shakti*. *Ida, Pingla* and *Sushumana Nadis* also meet at this chakra and form a Granthi. *Kundalini* energy is distinct from *prana* and sex energy. It is the creative power of God, kept in dormant state. Without the awakening of *Kundalini Shakti* the process of involution (journey of soul back to God) can never be started. The Muladhara chakra controls the excretory and sexual instinct functions in the body. This chakra corresponds with the *Bhu-Loka* (earth). Its Beej Mantra is LAM.

A yogi, who concentrates and meditates at this chakra acquire the full knowledge of the awakening of the Kundalini. When it is awakened, he gets the power (*siddhi*) to rise above from the ground (levitation). He is able to control his breath, mind and sex instinct. All his sins (fruits of past karmas) are destroyed, when the Kundalini enters his central *Brahma Nadi*. He acquires the knowledge of the past, present and future and becomes a *Trikala-Darsi*.

Remember:
"We are not alive only due to food and breath alone, but mainly due to the vital life force. We should try to know the technique to increase the reception of the life-force to develop & to vitalize our body-cells, mind, spirit and intuition."

"A deep & intense meditation activates the reception of the life force by medulla oblongata. The life force revitalizes the human body cells, the nerves and keeps all the body organs healthy & in perfect harmony with each other. The human body then functions in a better routine without any distortion & sickness. It keeps a firm control on the healthy development of body, mind, spirit and intellect."

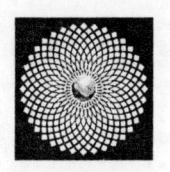

5

Asanas, Exercises, Mudras & Bandhas
for Awakening The Kundalini

Prayer
What are Asanas?
Sitting-Posture Asanas for Japa & Meditation
Selected Asanas More Useful for awakening the Kundalini
   Sarvangasana, Matsyasana (Fish Posture), Paschimottan-asana, Ardha-Matsyendra Asana, Vajra-Asana and Marudand-Asana, Shav-Asana (Corpse-Asana)

Some Useful Exercises (for Spine):
   Neck Rotation, Massage of the Scalp & Medulla Oblongata, Eyes Rotation Exercises

General Useful Instructions for Asanas & Pranayama

Mudras & Bandhas:
   Mula Bandha, Jalandhara Bandha, Uddiyana Bandha (Nauli Kriya), Maha-Mudra, Maha Bandha, Khechari Mudra, Shakti Chalana Mudra and Jyoti Mudra

Yoga is Equally Important for Women

Asanas, Exercises, Mudras & Bandhas for Awakening Kundalini

Prayer

O Divine Sea of Cosmic Life-Energy! Teach us how our five enchanting senses, our heart and digestive system are working continuously? Which energy is responsible for their continuous functioning? How can I be able to control my sense organs at my sweet will through Thy energy and will power? Teach me, why my body becomes tired during my awakening state, even if I do not work at all and take plenty of food to supply the physical energy to my body? And how my body is recharged again and becomes fresh during my sleep when I do not supply any physical energy to it through food?

O Sustainer of Life! Millions of complex chemical actions and reactions are always going on inside my body, even without my knowledge. No body is worried and responsible for all these actions & reactions, except Thee, not even my ownself. I bow to Thee.

What are Asanas?

Asanas: The Asanas are the different yogic postures, which helps in transmitting the life-energy, forcefully & willfully to different organs and nadis in the body. Through the special asanas yogis tries to stretch the particular organs of their body. By stretching the body the life-energy current flows vigorously in the stretched organ for a while. Then the whole body is relaxed to make the flow of life-energy normal.

Out of so many asanas, some of the asanas are more useful for curing the diseases, maintaining health and to awaken the Kundalini. An aspirant should preferably practice those asanas regularly. An aspirant may also practice some light exercises regularly along with the *yog-asanas*. These asanas and exercises promote and facilitate the flow of life energy in different parts of the body and make the breathing better. Asanas keeps our body free from diseases, keeps our health fit to meditate for a long time. Only a healthy body and healthy mind free from all kind of diseases can go to a state of deep meditation. A sick body and disturbed mind is unable to co-operate with the strain and stress of long meditation.

The cause of sickness and malfunctioning of some of the body organs is due to the lack of life force flowing in those body organs. The distribution of life force in the body is disturbed due to many habitual wrong postures and idleness. But by the *pranayama, asanas, mudras* and light exercises we try to send the life force, forcefully in every part of the body. The harmful bacterias, viruses and allergies are not able to affect a human body full of life force. Many advanced yogis have confirmed this fact scientifically, and remained unaffected by the bacterias and viruses.

There is a great misconception about yoga-asanas among most of the beginners, who think that *only the asana-*practice, is complete yoga. It is true that asanas are very important, to keep our body and mind healthy, and free from diseases. But the practice alone of some of the postures or asanas has nothing to do with the communion with God, which is the ultimate aim of Yoga. The *asanas* are enough to most of the persons in the world, who are only concerned to keep their physical body healthy and sound. But *asanas* alone are not enough for the seekers of God and Kundalini awakening. Many persons practice and teach some of the *asanas*, and claim themselves as a great yogi. They create a misconception about yoga. *Asanas* are only the third aphorism in the eightfold path of Patanjali *Yog-Sutras*.

Sitting Posture or Asanas For Meditation

There are four common asanas for Japa and Meditation. These are *Padmasana* (Lotus posture-crossed interlocked legs), *Siddhasana, Svastikasana* and *Sukhasana* (Easy posture-crossed legs). First put a soft cushion or a woolen blanket on a clean, secluded and lonely place on floor or hard bed in your house. Your body should be well insulated from earth. Some electric and life-energy current are generated during meditation. Your efforts will be wasted if these currents are earthed and are not insulated. While sitting in asana your spine, head and neck should erect upward. One should practice any one of above asana to sit at a stretch for hours. Padmasana is said to best, since your body cannot fall, even if you lost your body consciousness during meditation, but the Sukhasana is more comfortable and the easiest, if you do not lost body conscious while meditating.

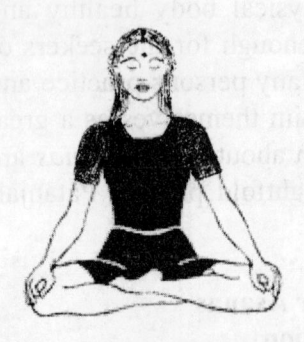

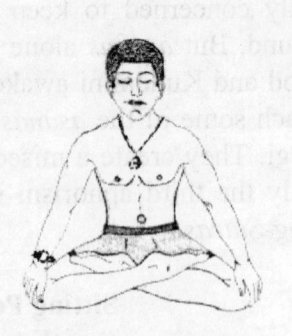

Sukhasana **Padmasana**

Stick to any one of the sitting asana you like. First watch your whole body and check internally. If there is any tension or a problem in any part of the body, relax that part to remove the tension. Then feel that you are sitting comfortably firm like a rock. You will soon get mastery on your asana for long meditation. The *asanas* gives strength and the *mudras* give a steadiness to the body.

Selected Asanas More Useful for Awakening the Kundalini

There are thousands of asanas and postures in all. Among these only few asanas are most useful, which will be describe here. Some of the asanas can be practiced in sitting, some in lying, some in standing and some in head downward-leg upward positions. Women should avoid the asana during their pregnancy.

These days many books are available especially on numerous asanas with illustrative pictures. But it is better to limit only to those asanas, which are more useful for deep meditation and awakening of the Kundalini.

1. Sarvang-asana & Hal-Asana

Both these asanas can be done simultaneously in one stretch. Spread a thick blanket on the clean floor. Lie down flat on your back. Slowly raise your legs vertically upward along with your trunk and hips. Support your back with your hands on either side. Rest your elbows on the ground. Press your chin against your chest, which is *Jalandhara Bandha*. Keep the legs straight & upward. Retain the breath as long as you can and slowly exhale through nose. When you are tired, either slowly brings down your legs to the ground or bend more your legs further like hal-asana. Remain in this posture for as much time as you can comfortably. Then bring back your legs and body to lie down flat on the floor. There should not any jerk while bringing up or down the legs. Then relax your whole body for a while with deep breath.

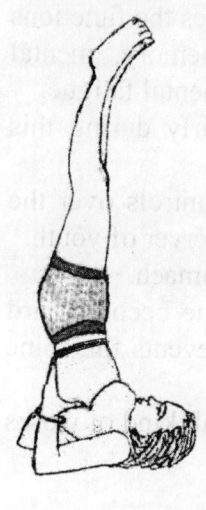

Sarvangasana

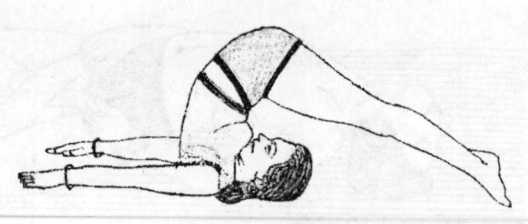

Hal-Asana (Plough-Asana)

In Sarvangasana your shoulders and elbows support the whole weight of the body. Do it only in the morning and the evening empty stomach. Along this asana *Hal-asana* can be done.

Benefits:
- Sarvangasana has all the benefits of *Sirshasana*. It is easier to do and has none of the risks of the *Sirshasana*.
- Since in these postures the head is at the lowest level of gravity, it supplies maximum amount of blood and prana to the brain to flow for a while. Consequently it relaxes & vitalizes the brain and removes many diseases connected with brain. It promotes the functions of the brain faculties. It increases memory, mental power and intelligence etc. It removes mental fatigue.
- You can hear the *Anahat* sounds clearly during this asana.
- It helps in maintaining celibacy and controls over the nightfall during dreams. So it is the preserver of youth.
- It eradicates diseases of intestine and stomach.
- In the old age the vertebras of the spine become hard and brittle known as ossification. It prevents the spine from early ossification (hardening).
- The lazy man becomes energetic to do all kind of works efficiently.

2. **Matsyasana (Fish Posture)**

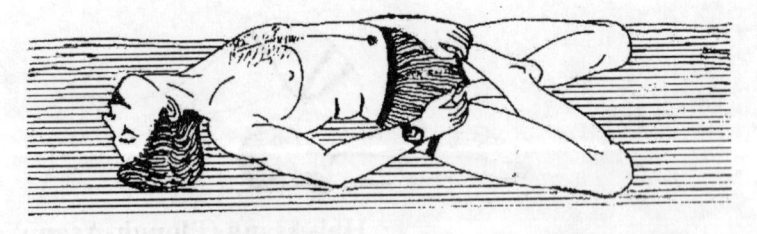

This asana should be practiced just after the Sarvangasana. It makes a man's body so light that he can float on water easily. This asana improves deep breathing.

Spread a woolen blanket on floor. Sit in Padmasana or Sukhasana with cross-legged. Lie down flat on the back. Hold the head up thus making the neck like an arch with the help of two elbows. Remain in this position for a comfortable duration of time. Then slowly release head with the help of hands and get up. Then unlock your legs. Take precaution of no jerk in spine, when you get up or lie down.

Benefits:
- Cures many diseases.
- It cures constipation and helps to ease out the faeces in the rectum.
- Useful in constipation, chronic bronchitis and asthma.

3. Paschimottan-Asana

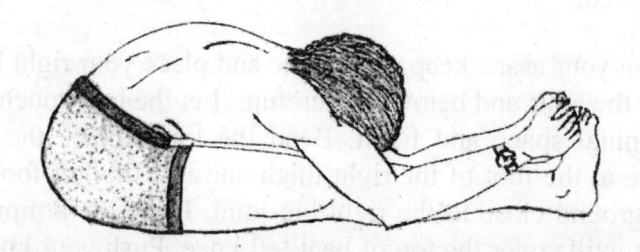

Sit on the blanket on the floor. Stretch both the legs flat like a stick. Bend the trunk forward slowly to catch your toes with the fingers and thumb. Try to touch your head with the knees. While bending exhale and retain the breath out for comfortable time. The spine of some may be hard and he may be not able to touch his head with the knees. He should not forcibly try to touch his head with the knees. It may take some time to get the success in this asana. Lift up the trunk and inhale a deep breath. Relax for a while. You should also repeat this asana with the stretching of only one leg and then reverse with the other leg.

Benefits:
- It activates the flow of prana in the *Brahma* Nadi *Sushumana* and stimulate in awakening the Kundalini.
- It increases the gastric fire.
- It reduces obesity and the enlarged spleen & liver.
- It stimulates the functioning of abdominal viscera, kidney, liver, dyspepsia and gastritis.
- It cures lumbago and myalgia, piles, prostate, lumber nerves epigastria plexus, bladder and diabetes etc.

4.   Ardha-Matsyendra Asana

In some of the asanas the trunk is bended forward and in some the trunk is bended backward. The trunk should also be twisted like a rope both clockwise and anticlockwise. Only then the perfect elasticity in the trunk can be achieved.

Sit on your asana keep erect spine and place your right heel near the anus and below the scrotum. Let the heel touch the perennial space and fix it. Bend the knee, place the left ankle at the foot of the right thigh and rest the left foot on the ground close to the right hip joint. Place the armpit or right axilla over the top of bent left knee. Push your knee a little to the back so that it touches the back part of the axilla. Try to catch the right palm with right foot. Apply a pressure at the right shoulder and slowly twist the spine to extreme left. Turn your face toward left. Try to retain this posture for a comfortable time.

Similarly you should reverse all the steps and twist your spine to the right side instead of left.

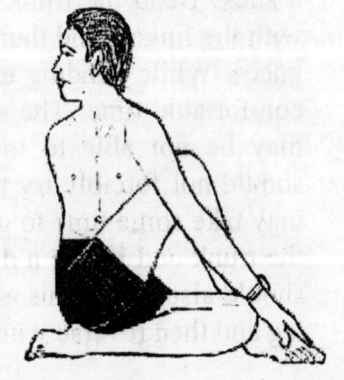

Benefits:
- This is an excellent and most useful asana, which helps in awakening of the Kundalini. It forces the flow of life-energy *in the Ida & Pingla Nadis*.
- It makes the spine elastic. All sorts of diseases like muscular rheumatism of the back, lumber spondylolysis and cervical etc. are cured.
- The spinal nerves and the sympathetic nervous system are toned up.

5. Vajra-Asana

This is a sitting pose asana, in which the trunk, spine and head are kept vertical. This is the only asana, which should be done just after taking the food. This asana stimulate the digestion of the food & you can sit in this asana for quite a long time. The legs are placed under the thigh. The soles are placed under the buttocks. The thighs must touch the calves. The whole weight of the body is put on the knees and the ankles. Keep hands gently on the knees. The knees are kept close to each other. Sit for as much time as you can in this asana.

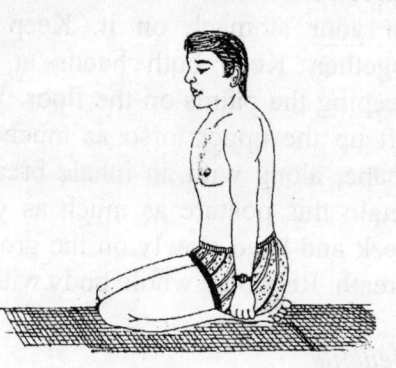

Benefits:
- Sciatica pain is cured.
- Flatulence is removed.
- The food is digested easily.
- The Myalgia in the knees, thighs, toes and legs is cured.
- It influences the *Kanda* from which all the Nadis spring and it is the most vital part of the body.

6. Bhujang-Asana (Snake-Asana)

The shape of this asana is just like snake that is why it is called as *Bhujang-Asana*.

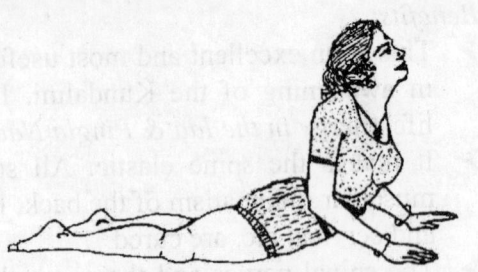

Spread a woolen blanket on the floor or hard bed. Lie down on your stomach on it. Keep the legs straight joined together. Keep both hands at the level of your chest keeping the palms on the floor. With the help of the arms, lift up the upper torso as much as you can do in an arc shape, along with an inhale breath. Hold your breath and retain this posture as much as you can. Lower the chest, neck and head slowly on the ground along with the exhale breath. Relax the whole body with deep breathing.

Benefits:
> It has all the benefits of **Paschimottan-Asana** as your spine bends in the opposite direction.

7. Dhanur-Asana (Bow-Asana)

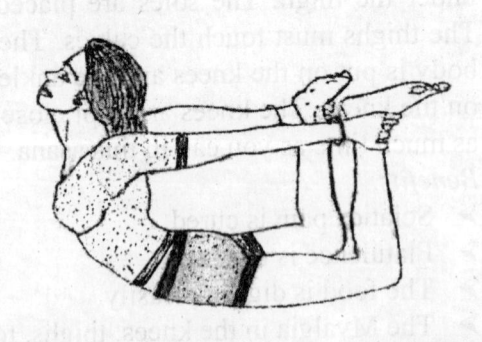

The shape of this asana is just like a bow (*Dhanush*). Lie down on your stomach on a woolen blanket on floor. Keep the legs straight and joined together. Bend your feet upward. Catch both the feet firmly with your both hands. Apply the force of stretching the arms & feet. Lift up your upper torso and the feet as much as you can in the arc shape along with a inhale breath. Hold the breath & retain the posture as much as you can. Slowly lower the chest; neck, head and your feet on the ground along with exhale breath. Relax the whole body with deep breathing.

Benefits:
➢ It has all the benefits of Bhujang-Asana and many more.

8. Marudand-Asana/ Exercises (for Spine)

This asana especially effects Spine, Ida, Pingla, and Sushumana. It is very useful to reduce the bulging stomach.

Stand straight. Lift your hands up along with breathing in. Bow down forward while breathing out, contract stomach inside and try to touch your feet. After a while stand straight up while breathing in. Then bend your spine backward as much as you can. Then bend forward backward. Repeat the same bowing backward, right side and left side. This is one cycle. Repeat as many cycles as you can. Then rotate your spine clockwise and anticlockwise, along with your hands keeping horizontally suspended.

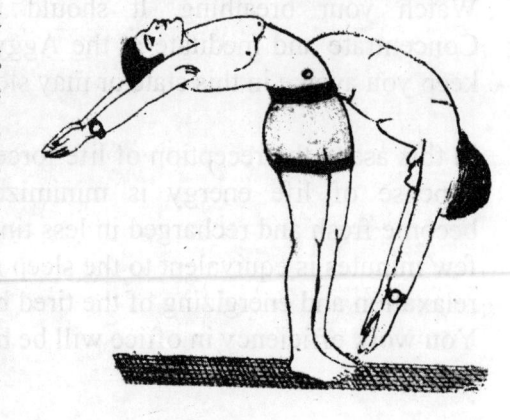

Benefits:
It has all the benefits of Bhujang-Asana and Dhanur-Asana.

9. Shav-Asana / Corpse-Asana

Shav-Asana is the most energizing and a useful Asana for the aspirants. It may be done in both the awakened and sleeping states and for as much time as you like. It is most simple also. This asana can be done at any time during the day even before your sleep.

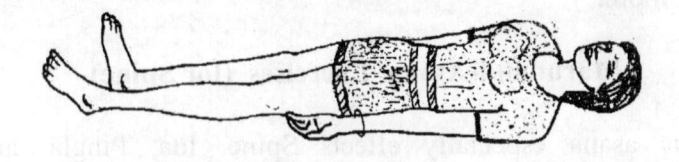

Shav-Asana

Lie down on flat on you back just as a corpse. Relax you whole body. Watch the tension if any, in each and every part of your body, starting from your feet. Relax the body part if you feel any tension there. While watching and starting from your feet lastly come to the Aggyia chakra. Watch your breathing. It should be deep and slow. Concentrate and meditate at the Aggyia chakra. You may keep you awake in this state or may sleep, as you like.

In this asana the reception of life force is increased and the expense of life energy is minimized. Your body will become fresh and recharged in less time. A Shav-Asana for few minutes is equivalent to the sleep for many hours in the relaxation and energizing of the tired body, brain and mind. You work efficiency in office will be better.

Some Useful Exercises

There is not much difference in slow exercises and the asanas. In the modern society most of us has to sit continuously on our chair or before a computer terminal in the office. Our neck and eyes remain in a fixed state, eyes looking and reading too much at a particular fixed position for most of the day. Most of us are straining our eyes and brain too much. If so, the following exercises should also be done.

1.   Neck Rotation Exercise:

Sit on your asana or stand vertical. Slowly rotate your neck clockwise and anticlockwise as many times as you like. Slowly move your neck upward and downward. Then slowly rotate the neck sideways, left and right. You may also do this exercise, in your office whenever you get a chance to do. It will cure and protect you from cervical.

2.   Hammering and Massage of the Scalp

Sit on your asana or stand vertical. Hammer your whole scalp slowly for a minute with your fists. Then massage the back of your neck at Medulla Oblongata with both the hands for some time. This will remove all the tiredness and tension due to excessive mental work. It will increase your memory and revitalize the brain cells.

3.   Eyes Rotation Exercises

Sit on your asana or stand vertical. Open your eyes and fix your neck. Rotate your eyes without the movement of your neck, clockwise and anticlockwise. Move your eyes upward, downward, sideways, and left & right as many times as you can. Your neck should not rotate or move while doing these exercises.

Stretch horizontal your right or left hand. Fix your eyes on the tip of your vertical thumb. Move your thumb horizontally closer and away to your eyes. These will certainly improve your eyesight and reduce the number of your specs.

General Useful Instructions for Asanas & Pranayama

- Be regular in practice.
- Take care of inhaling, exhaling and retaining your breath at the right moment during each asana.
- Initially one should learn the asanas from someone, who has already practiced.
- If japa is also done along with pranayama & asanas it will be better.
- The regular practice, patience and perseverance will give perfection in asanas & pranayama.
- Do not jerk and strain your body and spine more then your capacity. Perfection will come slowly.
- Keep remembering that the ultimate aim of asanas & pranayama is Self-Realization and awakening of the Kundalini and not simply to become healthy and cure diseases.

Mudras & Bandhas

The *Mudras* and *Bandhas* also play a vital role in the awakening of the Kundalini. *Gheranda Samhita* describes about 25 *mudras & bandhas*. But only seven are the most useful:

Asanas, Exercises, Mudras & Bandhas

1. Mula Bandha
2. Jalandhara Bandha
3. Uddiyana Bandha
4. Maha-Mudra & Maha-Bandha
5. Uddiyana (Flying)-Bandha
6. Khechari Mudra
7. Shakti Chalana Mudra

All the above mudras and bandhas are seldomly done separately. In most of the exercises, generally 2 or 3 mudras/ bandhas are combined with each exercise.

Benefits:
➤ Mudras & bandhas have all the benefits of the asanas & pranayama mentioned earlier.

1.   Mula Bandha

Press the yoni with the left heel. Keep the right heel pressed in the space just above the sex organs. Try to contract the anus upward and draw the *apana-prana* upwards. The apana-prana has the natural tendency to eject the excreta downwards. But in Mula Bandha we do just the opposite. We forcibly contract the anus upwards. In this practice both the prana & the apana-prana are forced to enter together in the Sushumana Nadi. Kundalini is awakened when the yogi achieves the perfection.

2.   Jalandhara Bandha

During pranayama after the deep inhalation, while holding the breath (*Kumbhak*), press your chin with the chest firmly. Retain comfortably as much as you can. This is known as Jalandhara Bandha.

3.   Maha-Mudra with Jalandhara-Bandha

Since it is the most useful it is called Maha (great) Mudra. Press the anus carefully with your right heel. Stretch out the left leg. Try to catch hold the toe with your hands. Inhale & hold your breath for a while. Then practice Jalandhara Bandha i.e. press your chin with the chest. Fix your concentration between at the Aggyia chakra. Try to remain in this posture as long as you can. Again reverse all the above steps. Relax.

4. Maha-Mudra & Maha-Bandha

➤ The practice of Maha-Mudra is necessary most useful before the fourteen Kriyas of Kriya-Yoga practice. It is very effective in straightening the spine and in the flow of proper distribution of life energy into spine and all parts of the body. It is done three times each in the morning and in evening.

➤ Sit with erect spine. Press the anus with the left heel. Draw the right leg up against the body, while inhaling slowly with a silent sound of 'Aaww…'. Retain and try to press the right leg towards chest with your interlocked fingers of hands.

➤ Feel a cool current is flowing upward from Muladhara to Aggyia chakra. Try to contract the anus and the muscles of the perineum upward. Try to draw apana-prana upwards. Exhale the breath with a inner sound of 'Eeeee..', bend the head down forward until the chin touches the chest.

➤ While holding the breath out stretch the right leg forward on the floor. Grasp the right foot with interlocked hands and try to touch your chin with your right leg.

- Sit up with inhaling breath with sound 'Aaaa..'. Make the spine erect with an exhaling slow breath with a mental sound of 'EEee'. Feel a hot current is flowing through the spine from Aggyia chakra to Muladhara chakra while exhaling.

- Repeat by reversing all the above steps by placing the left heel on the right thigh.

- Repeat all the above steps with both the legs drawn up against your body instead of one leg. Then stretch straight both the legs on the ground. The above three forms one cycle of Maha-Mudra. The cycle should be repeated three times.

- If you are not able to touch your chin with your legs flat on the floor, do not do it forcibly. You may get success after a few days of practice.

Maha-Mudra and Maha-Bandha stops the decay of body cells and preserves the youthfulness. It purifies Sushumana, Ida and Pingla nadis. Yogis achieve many Siddhis by this Mudra.

5. Uddiyana (Flying)-Bandha

Nauli Kriya (Pranayama) is the first stage of Uddiyana Bandha already explained in previous chapter. We completely empty the lungs forcibly with an exhale breath through the mouth. Then we contract and draw up the intestines above and below the navel toward the back. Then the abdomen rests firmly against the back of the body high up in the thoracic cavity. This is known as Uddiyana Bandha.

6. Khechari Mudra

Khechari means who can move in space. This Mudra can be learned only through an experienced expert guru who has already perfected it. It is difficult to master this Mudra. A qualified yogi cuts the lower tendon of the tongue of the yogi with a hygienic sharp blade. The cutting of the edges of tendon is done regularly more & more for a period of six months. The tongue is regularly massaged like the milking of the cow. By a regular practice the tongue is elongated so that its tip is able to touch the space between the eyebrows.

Sit on your asana. Touch the palate with your tongue and close the posterior nasal opening with the reversed tongue and fix your gaze on the Aggyia Chakra. It will activate the prana to flow in the Sushumana Nadi. By this way the tongue reaches the mouth of the well of nectar.

Although Khechari Mudra is said to be very useful, but I will not advise it, for all the aspirants, as it involves a risk of the damage of cutting the tendon of the tongue. You may avoid it and concentrate on others, which are equally useful.

Benefits:
> Yogi gets victory over many diseases, decay of body, old age and death. Yogi retains his youth for a long time. Yogi gets many *Siddhis*. Even the virulent poison may not harm him.

7. Shakti Chalana Mudra

Sit comfortably on your asana with erect spine. Inhale the air forcibly and combine it with the apana-prana. Do the Mula-Bandha and try to force the prana up into the *Sushumana* Nadi. Retain this position as long as you can.

You may feel the awakening of the Kundalini and trying to go up through the *Sushumana* Nadi.

Benefits:
➢ Helps in the activation of the awakening the Kundalini.

8. Jyoti Mudra

In Kundalini Yoga there is a great significance of third-eye or the single spiritual-eye in revealing the self or the Sprit. The realization of super and cosmic consciousness is possible only through meditation on single eye. This single-eye is visible easily through Jyoti mudra. It should be done just after your meditation. Practice:-

➢ Keep sitting in your meditation posture. Close each of the tragus (fleshy portion in front of the opening of the ear) of your ears with each of your hand thumb. Slightly press the outer corners of each of your closed eye with each of your index finger. Place the middle fingers on your nostrils and the forth fingers above your mouth. Place the little fingers below your mouth.
➢ Inhale with a sound of 'Aaww….' Assuming a cool current is flowing upward in the spine. Hold the breath while slightly pressing the eye corners. Concentrate at Aggyia chakra. The spiritual eye is visible.
➢ The spiritual eye may appear differently to different aspirants. Generally a revolving dark blue solid sphere of light surrounded by a hollow golden bright sphere of light is visible. A white five-pointed star is also visible at the centre of the blue disc.
➢ A Kriya-yogi has to concentrate and penetrate the white star seen at the centre of the spiritual third-eye. It represents the pure cosmic consciousness of the Absolute Brahman, who is beyond creation.

Yoga and Asanas are Equally Important for Women

It is illogical to say that yoga is only for men. God has given equal opportunity of self-realization to both men and women. Both have been provided with the dormant Kundalini Shakti to awaken it to achieve self-realization. Asanas are equally good for both men & women. Due to the advancement of science & technology so many modern machines are now available at homes for women, which have made their life more comfortable, easy and less time consuming. So now there is more necessity for Asanas, Pranayama and Exercises especially for women to keep themselves healthy and without obesity. Only during the pregnancy the women should avoid the asanas, but continue with light exercises and pranayama.

If the women learn the Asanas, Pranayam and Exercises they can easily transfer these to the younger children. It will keep them healthy and free from diseases. It will reduce the expense of great burden of providing free medical aids to its citizens by the Governments.

!Om Anandam Om!

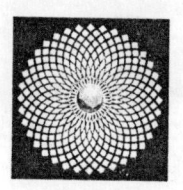

6

Purification of Body Nadis, Mind and Intellect

Prayer

Purification of Body, Nadis, Mind and Intellect

Some Useful Yoga Practices for Purification of Physical Body: *Dhauti, Basti, Jal-Neti, Nauli, Trataka, Kapalbha*ti

Pranayama Exercises:
1. Nadi Suddhi (purification of Nadis)
2. Sukha Purvaka (easy & comfortable) exercises.
3. Bhastrika
4. Ujjayi
5. Suryabhedi
6. Plavini
7. Pranic Healing (The Secret of Reiki)
8. The Distance Pranic Healing (Reiki)

6
Purification of Body Nadis, Mind and Intellect

Prayer

O Cosmic Father! O Divine Mother of Creation! Teach me to understand Thy secret of creation. O Cosmic Mother! Teach me to heal from the various diseases of my physical body, by recharging it with Thy cosmic life energy. Make me realize Thy presence beneath the waves of the creation. Thou art constantly working and arranging the atoms, molecules and the subatomic particles to create the living cells, organs and bodies. The living cells are further being arranged themselves as building blocks of matter inside the living bodies. Thou art secretly controlling the growth of trillions of living bodies? Reveal Thy Knowledge of creation and controlling.

Purification of Body, Nadi Mind & Intellect

There are many kinds of yogas prevalent among the aspirants. But the different yogas cannot be separated in the watertight compartments. So a harmonious combination of all the yogas is necessary for the easy and fastest awakening of the Kundalini. It is agreeable by all that before awakening the *Kundalini* the aspirants should purify their Physical Body, Nadis, Mind and Intellect. Otherwise the aspirant may face some uncontrollable problems beyond the understanding and cure by the medical doctors.

Useful Yoga Practices for the Purification of Physical Body

The purification of physical body by an aspirant can be achieved by the following six yogic exercises. Dhauti, Basti, Neti, Nauli, Trataka and Kapalbhati. These are known as six Sat-Karmas of Hath Yoga and should be practiced daily.

(1) Dhauti Kriya

Dhauti kriya is of many types:
A – *By a muslin cloth:* It is done with the help a 3" wide and 15' long clean hygienic muslin cloth free from germs & bacterias. The yogi swallows the cloth slowly and takes it out slowly. Both the food pipe and the stomach are being well cleaned by this kriya. The muslin cloth is being well washed with soap after the kriya.

B - *Kunjal Kriya*: Drink a large quantity of pure water at normal temperature when the stomach is empty in the morning. Retain it comfortably for some time. Contract the stomach and vomit the water out completely. This kriya cleans the stomach; improve the digestion and removes acidity.

C – Teeth, Tongue and Eyes Cleaning: Teeth, tongue and eyes are cleaned by any suitable, conventional and convenient method every day by the yogis.

(2) Basti Kriya

Jal (water)-Basti or Anima Kriya: Instead of actual Jal-Basti done by the yogis, I would suggest the alternative comfortable anima kriya, which is easy and less time consuming. The Naturopathy doctors also frequently use it. Take nearly one kg of luke-warm pure water in the anima pot easily available with the chemists. Put a small quantity of common salt or limejuice into it. The anima kriya cleans the deposits and worms etc inside the anus, large and small intestine of the man. The digestive system is improved and so many diseases connected with the digestive system are cured.

(3) Jal-Neti Kriya
(Cleaning nostrils and throat with water)

In Jal-Neti kriya the nostrils and throat are cleaned with luke-warm saline water. The Jal (water)-Neti kriya is very easy and very useful. Jal-Neti does not require any specialized training. A special type of water-pot like small tea-cattle is used for Jal-Neti kriya.

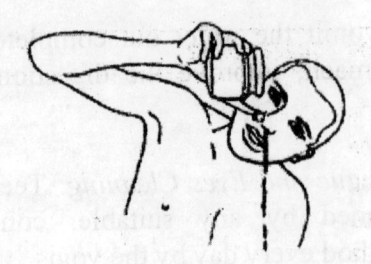

Jal-Neti Kriya

The luke-warm hygienic saline water is sucked by one of the nostril and is expelled from the other nostril and the mouth simultaneously. A continuous flow of water stream is maintained through the nostrils. The flow of water in the nostrils is reversed, after half of the process. After the Neti expel forcefully all the remaining water inside the nostrils. A few drops of pure ghee (butter oil), olive oil or coconut oil may be put in the nostrils at the end.

After the cleaning of the nostrils the breathing becomes regular and deep. It is a sure shot cure for all type of colds, bronchitis and asthma without any medicine.

(4)   Nauli Kriya

This kriya is intended for regenerating, invigorating and stimulating the abdominal viscera and the gastro-intestinal system. For Nauli the practice of Uddiyana Bandha is needed. Nauli is generally done in the standing position with empty stomach.

I. First stand up with your legs apart. Rest your hands downwards on your thighs. Forcibly exhale your breath out through your mouth so that your stomach is completely empty of air.

II. Forcibly contract the stomach and the abdominal muscles so that the wall of the stomach is stretched backwards. This is known as Uddiyana Bandha the first stage of Nauli.

III. Now try to contract the muscles of your stomach in the centre, or at right or at left side and try to rotate the abdominal muscles. Do this practice slowly and progressively. You will learn it within few weeks. Beginners may feel it little difficult with slight pain in the initial practice. Do not be afraid of this practice. The liver and pancreas are toned up by this practice.

(5) *Trataka* Kriya (Continuous Gazing)

Trataka kriya is the process of continuously gazing at a fixed point without winking the eyes. Trataka is necessary and useful to learn the art of concentration and meditation.

To practice it: Fix your eyes at a point or a bright object or on a candle flame or on the picture of the god you have a faith, placed at a distance of nearly 3 feet at the level of your eyes. Gaze it continuously without winking the eyes. Be firm and steady till your eyes begin to flow the tears. Then close your eyes and visualize the same mentally inside.

You may also concentrate on a bright star or moon at night, or just at blank sky during the day or any particular color you like. You may look at the image of your pupils continuously in front of a plane mirror.

Advanced students can do *Trataka* at the inner chakras in the spinal cord. This Trataka can be done even during the walk or traveling in a vehicle. The duration of Trataka is gradually increased. During Trataka the mind is kept peaceful under control. Trataka at Aggyia Chakra (the space between two eye brows) is most useful. Trataka improves your eyesight. The number of the spectacles is reduced. The will-power and mental-power are increased. Memory becomes sharp and one takes less time to study the same. One can achieve educational higher aims easily.

Trataka is different from concentration. The practice of *Trataka* helps in the concentration of mind on a single thought. The regular practice of concentration further helps in the practice of deep meditation. A long meditation is necessary to awaken the Kundalini and to experience *samadhi*.

6. *Kapalbhati*

Kapalbhati is one of the six purification exercises for the purification of the skull and lungs. It is a kind of pranayama exercise. It is similar to *Bhastrika* pranayama with a minor difference.

Sit in any comfortable asana like *Padmasana* (cross interlocked legs) or *Siddhasana* or *Sukhasana* (easy crossed legs). Keep your hands on your knees. Perform inhalation (*puraka*) and exhalation (*rechaka*) rapidly in a cycle. Make puraka (retaining breath) little long and mild and make *rechaka* quick and forcible. There is no retention of breath (*Kumbhak*) at the end. The exhalation should be done quickly and forcibly. This is one cycle. One should gradually increase the number of cycles of this pranayama.

In *Bhastrika* pranayama there is retention of breath at the end of the practice. Both the puraka and rechaka are done equally quickly. This is the only difference between the two.

Kapalbhati cleanses both the respiratory system and the nasal passages. It cleanses and removes the spasm from the bronchial tubes. Consequently bronchitis & asthma are cured by regular practice. Both the blood circulatory system and the respiratory systems are purified and toned up. Consequently all the diseases connected with the two are cured.

Nadis are also purified and affected by the pranayama. Kundalini energy cannot pass through the impure nadis. If awakened, it will either create problems or it will go to dormant state again. So it is necessary first to purify the nadis with pranayama.

Pranayama

Pranayama is the science of controlling the omnipresent cosmic life force through the special exercises of controlling the breath. Breath is directed forcibly by our mind under the control of our will. It is a vitalizing, regenerated force, which can be utilized consciously for our spiritual development and for the healing of the incurable diseases.

If we are able to control the prana energy associated through our breath, chakras, nadis and mind then the secret of subjugating the prana will be known to us. The mastery over the universal prana energy gives a victory over all kind of fear. An attractive aura is developed around the yogis, which influence others. They become more fascinating and charming.

Our soul is covered with three *gunas* known as *rajas, tamas* and *satwik*. The rajas & tamas gunas are removed by the pranayama exercises. Pranayama purify our body, mind, nadis and intellect.

Pranayama is related with our breath and thoughts. By the control of breath we can control the prana flowing in our body and by controlling the prana we can control our five sense organs, thoughts and mind. Our breath is the flywheel of the engine of pranayama controlling our body. If we can control the flywheel we can control all the moving parts of machinery.

By the control of mind, yogi can control his instinct of sex, anger, pride, greed and attachments. Just similar to our physical body we have an astral body overlapping with each other. There are networks of overlapping similar nerves & Nadis in both the bodies. Prana flows in the both the networks of Nerves of physical & Nadis of astral bodies. There is an intimate connection and interaction between the pranas flowing in two systems.

Pranayama Exercises

There are many varieties of pranayam exercises. One may chose the exercises suitable to one's temperament, characteristics and constitution. It is not necessary to do all the exercises at a time daily. Pranayama should be done early in the morning and in the evening after the nature calls. It is better, if pranayama is done in the open air or well-ventilated room in a lonely and peaceful place. It requires a deep concentration and empty stomach. A *japa* of Aum mantra along with Pranayama is better.

Pranayama are mainly the deep breathing exercises:
1. Nadi Suddhi (purification of Nadis)
2. Sukha Purvaka (easy & comfortable) exercises

3. Bhastrika
4. Ujjayi
5. Suryabhedi (& Jalandhara Bandha)
6. Plavini
7. Pranic Healing

Nadi-Suddhi Pranayama
(Pranayama for Purification of Nadis)

This pranayama should be done first. The purification of nadis is the main consideration in the early stages of Kundalini yoga. If the nadis are impure the ascent of Kundalini is blocked in the Sushumana. Purity of the nadis facilitates the ascent of Kundalini without any trouble. The daily Nadi-Suddhi pranayama practice quickly purifies the nadis.

The aspirant sits in any comfortable asana such as *Padmasana or Siddhasana or Sukhasana* with erect spine and relaxed body. First, one should offer prayers to Guru & God. Then concentrate at the point between the eyebrows. Close the right nostril with your right thumb. Then inhales through *Ida* (left nostril) for 16 counts, retain for 64 counts and exhale through *Pingla* (right nostril) for 32 counts. Then reverse the kriya, inhale through Pingla for 16 counts, retain for 64 counts and exhale through Ida for 32 counts. It is one cycle. It is repeated five times. Instead of counting one may practice japa with *Beej* mantra.

Sukha Purvaka Pranayama

Sit in any asana with erect spine and relax body. Close the right nostril with your right thumb. Inhale a deep breath with your left nostril and whisper Om sound 3 times.

Concentrate your attention on the air you are breathing in. Feel that you are drawing in the cosmic prana energy with air. Then retain the breath inside by closing your left nostril by your little finger till 12 counts of Oms. Then imagine that you are forcibly sending the prana current striking at the Muladhara Chakra to awaken the Kundalini sleeping there.

Open the right nostril and exhale through the right nostril for 6 counts of Oms, keeping close the left nostril. The time ratio for inhale: retain: exhale is 1:4:2. You may increase the time and counts of whispering Oms in retaining the breath, but it should be comfortably without any strain to lungs and without any hurry.

It will be better for awakening the Kundalini, if the aspirant contracts up the anus nerves. It is known as Mula Bandha. Concentrate at the Kundalini sleeping in Muladhara. A deep concentration and strong will to awaken the Kundalini always helps. This pranayam should be practiced daily & regularly.

Benefits:
- Purifies Nadis.
- Removes all diseases.
- Improves blood circulation and digestion.
- Helps in controlling sex instinct, mind, and awaken the Kundalini.

Bhastrika Pranayama

Bhastrika means bellows, breathing rapidly just as a blacksmith blows his bellows rapidly. In the similar way one has to breath in and out rapidly. Sit comfortable in any asana with erect spine. Close your mouth. Inhale and exhale forcibly and rapidly 20 times like the bellows.

Constantly dilate your lung at inhale and contract your lung at exhale repeatedly. Start with a forcibly expulsion of air, inhale and again exhale forcibly and repeatedly. Concentration on exhale; inhale and retain will be automatically.

At the end when you are tired, inhale a deep breath and retain it comfortably for as much time as you can and then you exhale slowly. Rest for a while after one round and enjoy the peace inside. This is one cycle of the exercise. Increase your rounds from 3 to 20 gradually but comfortably. Bhastrika can be done even in standing position.

Benefits:
- Reduces phlegm and cure asthma and all the disease of nose, lungs and throat inflammation.
- Improves digestion, eradicates asthma and the diseases concerning with excess of gas and bile.
- It produces warmth in the body.
- Bhastrika enables the prana to flow forcibly in three main Granthis in the Chakras, through which the Kundalini has to pierce.

Ujjayi Pranayama

Sit in your comfortable asana with erect spine. Inhale slowly a deep breath from both the nostrils with sound of 'So' and expand your chest. Retain your breath as long as you can comfortably. Then exhale the breath slowly from your left nostril by closing the right nostril with your right thumb with a sound of 'Ham'. A peculiar sound is produced while inhaling. Repeat it 5 to 10 times.

Benefits:
- It cools the head. Gastric fire is increased.

- Removes asthma & phlegm in nose & throat.
- Pulmonary diseases are cured.
- Protect us from enlargement of spleen, dyspepsia, dysentery and cough etc.

Suryabhedi Pranayama & Jalandhara Bandha

Sit comfortably in any asana with erect spine. Close your eyes. Close the left nostrils with your right ring and little fingers. Inhale slowly through the right nostril as long as you can, without making any sound. Close both the nostrils with your fingers and retain the breath firmly by pressing your chin against the chest. This is known as (*Jalandhara Bandha*). Try to hold your breath till the perspiration oozes from the roots of the body hairs. Heat is produced in the body by this pranayama. You may not get success in the first instant, but try to increase the time for holding your breath. You will get success.

Benefits:
- It purifies the brain and destroys the intestinal worms.
- It cures all diseases caused due to gas (vayu) and rheumatism.
- It cures rheumatism and all sorts of neuralgia. The sinus infection is also cured.

Plavini Pranayama

It is little difficult pranayama. The yogi sits in asana & drinks the air like water and fills the stomach like an expended balloon. The body becomes light, due to increase of volume and may float on water. At the end air is exhaled slowly.

The Pranic Healing Pranayama
(The Secret of Reiki)

By the continuous practice of the pranayama exercises and other aphorism of yoga one can impart his pranic energy to others for the healing of their morbid diseases. The advanced aspirants (*sadhaks*) can recharge their bodies with prana energy and are able to transfer the same to the diseased man. One should not be afraid and think that his own pranic energy will be depleted due to the distribution of life energy to others. Rather it will flow more through him, as the knowledge never decreases by distributing it to others. This is a spiritual law.

Before practicing this technique on others, one should learn first to direct his own pranic healing energy to his own diseased part of the body. Most of our diseases are simply due to the lack of the pranic-energy flowing in the diseased part. But by our strong will and regular practice it is possible to send and direct the pranic-energy to flow in any organ of our body. When one gets mastery over his own body, then he may apply it to others.

Hiranyagarbha is the cosmic source (ocean) of pranic-energy. Suppose you have a sluggish kidney and want to cure it. Sit comfortably on your asana. Do Nadi Suddhi & Sukha Purvaka pranayama. Close your eyes. Concentrate on *Hiranyagarbha* to charge your body fully with pranic-energy. Then direct the pranic-energy to flow in your kidney. Concentrate and fix your mind at the diseased part (kidney) for some time. Then by your strong will power direct the prana to penetrate the tissues of kidney.

During the exhalation of breath imagine that all the diseases are flowing out through your breath. Repeat it 10 times. Since the pranic-energy has got infinite intelligence to cure, to repair the tissues and do the regenerative microscopic constructive works; therefore the disease part will be cured. Pranic healing may not be instantaneous it may take few days to cure a disease.

By the regular practice of pranayama and asanas a yogi simply send the mysterious life-energy forcibly to all the different organs of his body. This keeps the physical body of the yogi healthy free from all diseases. A yogi need not run after the allopathic doctors and medicines for day today heath problems. The natural herbs and pranic-energy-healing (Naturopathy) are the best gifts of God given to humanity to keep itself healthy.

If some body is suffering with lack of life-energy in his diseased organ, an advanced yogi may help him to provide the life-energy. He charges his body with the life-energy by pranayama, by concentrating at *Hiranyagarbha*. Then he should touch or massage the diseased organ of the patient. Then he should imagine that the cosmic energy is flowing through his hands to the diseased organ of the patient. The life-energy will obey him and the patient will be cured in few days.

Distant Pranic Healing
(Reiki)

The advanced yogis can cure others from a distance also. It is not necessary that the yogi and the patient should be in close bodily contact. But the patient must have a firm faith and a positive attitude both in the power of healing by life-energy and the yogi who is doing it.

The yogi should inform the patient to sit comfortably and close his eyes at a particular time on a particular date. The patient should also imagine that he is receiving the pranic-energy from the yogi, to cure his diseased organ at that particular time. The yogi should do his *Kumbhak* pranayama (retention of breathing) at the right appointed time. The yogi should mentally direct the pranic-energy, to transmit it to the patient through the space. He should imagine that the energy is penetrating in the diseased organ of the patient. Yogi may recharge himself again & again with pranic-energy through *Hiranyagarbha* which travels like the radar or laser waves in the space. For any kind of waves, there must be a transmitter and receiver. Here the transmitter is yogi and the receiver is patient. Similar is the pranic healing practice.

General Benefits of Pranayama

- Helps in awakening the Kundalini.
- Enable to listen the Anahat sounds.
- Eyes sparkles like diamonds.
- Body becomes strong, healthy, lean and free from diseases.
- Voice becomes sweet and melodious.
- Celibacy is achieved.
- Victory over anger, greed, proud and attachments is achieved.
- Nadis are purified.
- Happiness & peace is achieved.
- Victory over fear of future uncertainty is achieved.
- Victory over *Rajas & tamas gunas* is achieved.
- The diseases connected with the breathing are cured.

!Om Anadam Om!

We must have clear understanding and a strong will power to control our mental emotions, discrimination between right & wrong, or good & bad actions. Only our right & pure thoughts and feelings can bring us the greatest happiness and joy in life."

"If you don't invite God to be your summer Guest, He will not come to you in the winter of your life."

"Seek divine eternal wealth & not the perishable paltry tinsel of earth."

!Om Anandam Om!

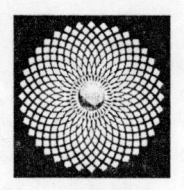

7

Techniques of Awakening The Kundalini

Prayer

The Necessity of a Spiritual Guru

Kundalini Shakti is the Spiritual Energy for Involution

Relation of a Yogi with God

What Happens during the Meditation?

Concentration is Different from Meditation

When and How to Meditate?

Meditation Technique of Awakening Kundalini useful for a Kriya Yogi

Listening & Meditation on Anahata Sounds (Laya Yoga) or *Surat-Shabda* Yoga for a Kriya Yogi

Bhakti Yoga: The Yoga with Devotion & Worshipping of God

Kriya Yoga Technique of Awakening Kundalini

7
Techniques of Awakening The Kundalini

Prayer

O Cosmic Mother! Teach me to heal from various diseases of my physical body, by recharging it with Thy cosmic life energy. Make me realize Thy presence beneath the waves of creation. Thou art constantly working and arranging the atoms, molecules and the subatomic particles to create the living cells. By Thy intelligence the living cells are further being arranged as building blocks of organs inside the living bodies.

O, *Omnipresent Cosmic Sound of Aum,* open my sixth sense of intuition, to know thy secret of creation, savoir and destruction of the universe. Thou art creating & rearranging the five gross elements. These five gross elements again dissolve into thy Cosmic Sea at the end of the universe. Heavenly Father! Make me understand and realize Thy secret of *creation, preservation and annihilation.* Tell me my insignificant role to play in thy divine universal drama of cosmic dream. Reveal Thyself.

Necessity of a Spiritual Guru

A Guru is one who is self-realized, enlightened and is able to remove the veil of ignorance or *Maya* in his deluded disciples. A Guru is Truth, Brahman, Atman, God and beyond the strong bond of *Maya*. He must have experienced the enlightenment after the awakening of his Kundalini. A Guru has an unconditional love with his disciples.

The grace of both the God and a Guru is needed to awaken the Kundalini and to merge it up with Lord Shiva sitting in Sahasrara. A guru is a guide, a searchlight and the spiritual preceptor & motivator in the unknown inner journey of the soul back to merge in God. A Guru is Brahman & God Himself. The service of Guru is the service of God. The mere presence of Guru works as a catalyst for soul in elevating, inspiring, self-illuminating and the Guru's words are the words of Brahman. A highly learned man cannot be called a Guru, if he is not enlightened.

A real Guru may have the power to awaken the Kundalini of his disciples through a simple touch, or a mantra, or a mercy gaze or in so many other ways he likes. This is known as **Shaktipat**. But the Guru should always avoid *Shaktipat* in his disciples. It is always better if the Kundalini is awakened automatically through the own yogic efforts of a disciple, after his body is fully purified and becomes fit for the immense energy released by the Kundalini. If the Kundalini is prematurely awakened in a non-purified body it may lead to waste and some uncontrollable problems may arise unknown by the doctors and the Guru.

Kundalini Shakti is the
Spiritual Energy for Involution
(The Journey of Soul - Back to God)

The *Kundalini Shakti* is different from the primary life force or the *Prana Shakti*. It is sleeping in dormant form at the *Muladhar chakra*. It is the Creative Intelligent Force of God. It is also known as the *'Voice of Silence'*. By regular practice of *Yog-Sutras* and intense devotion to God, one day *Kundalini Shakti* is awakened by the grace of God on yogi. The yogis generally experience it as a snake sleeping in two & half round at *Muladhar Chakra*.

The Kundalini power is just similar to the creative cosmic power of God hidden in the dormant form inside all the seeds. The future birth and development of the whole tree is already hidden in a seed like a hidden computer software program in the hard-disc (seed). But the seed is not aware of his hidden energy and the hidden program. When a farmer puts the seed into moist soil at a favorable temperature and environment, the dormant creative energy of the seed is awakened and begins to work inside. The seed is sprouted; its old body dies and took a new birth in a new body as a plant. After few days there is no trace of the original seed in the plant. Even then everything goes on progressing exactly the same, as hidden inside the original seed. Where and how does this program is preserved inside the seed and the tree is a mystery?

The above example is similar to the Kundalini power hidden in dormant form inside man. Man is not aware of this hidden energy. Like farmer a realized Guru helps in creating the proper psychological and environmental conditions for the awakening of the Kundalini power of his disciple. When it awakens, there is a new inner birth of the

aspirant and at the same time it is also the death of his previous personality. In case of man it is not visible as a physical change in his body unlike that of seed, but it is a complete inner astral change in the perception of his soul, body and the concept of the universe and God. There are two types of Kundalini Shakti in human:
1. *Individual* Kundalini Shakti
2. *Universal* Kundalini Shakti

The *Individual Kundalini Shakti* is the divine liquid fire that rushes up through the innermost core of spine known as *Sushumana* and pierces through the six *Chakras* one by one. *Ida, Pingla and Sushumana* are the three main *Nadis* in our subtle body. Without the awakening of this *Kundalini* power no subtle spiritual experience or *Samadhi* is possible. The Individual Kundalini Shakti is different in different man but has connection with the Universal Kundalini Shakti, which is one throughout.

The *Universal Kundalini Shakti* is said to be the cosmic force, power or energy of the divine that created the universe and it is constantly evolving and developing new materials, atomic and sub-atomic particles and their different forms. It is a single energy working throughout the universe. It has a creative and imaginative power along with intelligence.

Generally the *Individual Kundalini Shakti* is spontaneously awakened with the grace of God and due to the own efforts of the aspirant. If Kundalini is forcibly awakened without prior purifying of the body, mind and spirit, it may give some trouble to the yogi. If the *sushumana* in the spine is not ready for it, then its huge mysterious power of high voltage becomes uncontrollable by the yogi. The risk is less if it rushes straight upward without any blockade in

Techniques of Awakening The Kundalini

Sushumana Nadi, but more if it turns downwards or sideways.

A yogi should not be afraid of awakening of his *Kundalini,* if he is practicing and following all the *Yog-Sutras* properly. The process of involution (the journey back to God) and spiritual unfoldment starts only after the awakening of the *Kundalini Shakti. Kundalini* is an initiation for entry into the ocean of divine knowledge. As the *Kundalini* crosses the *Chakras* one by one, there are some subtle inner experiences of other worlds to the yogi and he achieves many *siddhies* (divine miraculous powers and knowledge). No self-realization is possible without the awakening and rushing up the *Chakras* by the *Kundalini Shakti and merging in Sahasrar.* Without awakening of his *Kundalini Shakti* and raising it upto *Sahasrar* there can't be any spiritual *Guru.*

Except the man, none of the living being, including the deities have been provided the individual Kundalini Shakti for their salvation. This means none other then man can get self-realization. If a deity wants to get self-realization, he will have to take a birth in the human form.

Relationship of a Yogi with God

It is important for a yogi to have a relation (bond of love) with God. A yogi can have any relation with God like: Lord-bhakta, Father-son, Friend-friend, Swami-disciple or the aspirant is one with God. If the aspirant has no relation with God, his bond of love with God will be weak. A yogi is not a physical body, but simply an *Atma* (soul) and God is *Paramatma* (supreme soul). Both do not posses any physical body and therefore have no sex concept. The sex is related with the physical body and not the characteristic of the soul. Our soul is neither a male nor a female.

Most of the yogis develop the following relations with God: Divine Father--son; Divine Mother--son; Supreme Lover--beloved; Lord—servant (das); *Paramatma--atma*; Swami--disciple; Friend—friend; God--*gopika*; God and ego 'I' are one and the same (*'So-Ham', or 'Aham Brahmashmi', or 'Tatvamasi'*) etc. The relation may not be fixed or permanent throughout the life of the yogi. Generally it changes from time to time.

What Happens During Meditation

"Meditation is the cessation of the mind from all thoughts for a long time." Meditation is an effort of a yogi, by his constant practice to realize and express that the pure consciousness is the reflection of God within you. Meditation is the joyful state of mind, when it is perfectly tuned with God.

After a fixed concentration of mind for a long duration, mind becomes thoughtless but with awareness of ego 'I'. In this state, mind is undisturbed by the five senses and distracting stray thoughts of the outer enchanting world. Mind is totally interiorized. Our body consciousness is forgotten. We forget about all the demands and the necessities of the physical body. But we are aware of our ownself. Meditation is the dieing process of a yogi to the world without actually dieing of the body. Remember we should not sleep during meditation. During meditation we are neither in this world nor in the sleep-world.

During meditation we are able to stop our thoughts consciously, what we do unconsciously every night to sleep. One experiences oneness with God along with bliss and joy. During meditation the heartbeats become slow and BP is lowered. Distracting senses are cut off from the mind. The outer disturbances like noise, smell, touch, taste and vision does not disturb the yogi as in the sleeping state senses do not disturb. The yogi's mind becomes like an undisturbed peaceful pond of still water. Breathing becomes deep and slow. Pulse rate is decreased. Body organs start feeling like dead one by one. The digestive system is slowed down. The expense of life energy by different organs of the body becomes negligible. The reception of life energy by the medulla oblongata increases many folds. Tired body cells begin to recharge, by the life force. The life force begins to repair the diseased parts of the body.

Concentration is Different From Meditation

The word concentration has come from concentric circles, which have common centre. Fixing of mind on one object or one thought is known as concentration. It is the tendency of the naughty mind to switch over to different thoughts and objects. A yogi tries to tame and fix his mind on a single thought. If it distracts to other thoughts, bring it back to the original thought. If your mind is able to fix on one object or a single thought for long, you are in a state of concentration. It is just like the poring of oil from one bottle to another. Remember; during concentration one should not sleep, but keep awaken continuously.

Now try to get away with the single thought or object of concentration and become thoughtless and objectless. Mind should become blank free from all kinds of thoughts. It is now the meditation state. Your mind becomes thoughtless but with awareness of ego 'I'. You are neither sleep nor awake, but in between the two states. It is known as the *'Turia-avashatha'* (a state of pure consciousness).

"God has fixed our consciousness to face and look outward. Therefore, the ordinary mortal men gazes outward, but a few desiring immortality or to know self, turn the gaze inward and see the self and God within".
- Katha Upanishad

There are only two things: 'The world' and 'the God'. Human beings are placed between the two. Other creatures have no concept of God. We feel pleasures by coming in contact with the enchanting worldly things through our senses and develop attachment with them. But a yogi realizes that the bliss and joy in meditation is much more enchanting than all the worldly pleasures. Due to the great impact of *Maya* we generally avoid doing experiment with God, because we have neither tasted nor have the knowledge of God. None has helped us in developing the devotion and love for God. *If only once we are able to experience the eternal bliss and the joy of God, we will always hanker after it for the rest of our life.* One should not doubt on it.

During meditation visualize that the cosmic life-energy is entering our body through the medulla oblongata at the centre of the skull. This life energy is directed to the *Aggyia Chakra*, which distributes it to other *Chakras* in the *Sushumana*, which further distribute it to different body organs to function.

Techniques of Awakening The Kundalini   147

Try to *interiorize your mind, look within yourself.* Presume that infinite God is everywhere around you. Try to merge your consciousness into super-consciousness. You can transcend your mind through eternity and can go beyond the galaxies. Try to listen to God's voice. Whenever we make a mistake, God warns us silently. If we ignore His voice, He becomes quite. But when we pay attention to listen to Him, He will guide us. By constantly following His voice, we will be transformed into a peaceful, truly moral person.

Remember that all the thoughts are coming from God and are stored in the ocean of ether. God knows the course of all our thoughts. Unless and until we *completely surrender* ourself to God, God will not like to reveal Himself to us. When we surrender all our worldly desires to God, God blesses us. You may be very busy throughout the day and much tired, even then never go to bed, without the deepest attention & meditation on God.

Due to the power of *Maya* we perceive ourself as a body consisting flesh, bones and nerves. This is the cause of our many troubles and sorrows in the world. If we meditate continuously and unceasingly, we can quickly realize that we are not the physical body but the infinite essence of God. We will be free from all our problems, miseries, pains and sorrows. It will also make us free from the bondage of our physical body.

When and How to Meditate?

Since the digestion becomes slow during the meditation, it should be done only when the stomach is empty. The best times are early morning, evening, just before lunch or dinner, and just before sleep. During meditation some electricity is generated in the body, so the yogi should sit, on an insulated, soft and comfortable cushion to cut off the body currents from earth. There should be regularity of practice and time everyday. During meditation one must have deep devotion for God. Without devotion the achievement is less and useless. Ask your family members not to disturb you by anybody and even by a radio, T.V., phone or doorbell etc. during your meditation time.

Practice: Select a remote, clean, airy and beautiful place in your house for daily meditation at fixed timings. Since the earth magnetic field and rotation has an effect on the mind, it is better to face towards North or East in meditating posture. Sit on a clean, soft and comfortable cushion placed on floor. The cushion helps to keeps the body cut-off from the heat and electric currents from earth, produced in the body during meditation. You may sit, crossed-legged in a comfortable posture (*Sukhasana*) or in *Padmasana* posture. For short meditation simple crossed legged *Sukhasana* is sufficient, but for longer meditation *Padmasana* is better, which prevents the body from falling.

➢ First watch the inside & outside of body thoroughly. If there is any tension in any part of the body relax it. Next lightly close the eyes to cutoff the light distractions of the outer world. Again watch your body thoroughly. If still there is any tension in any part of the body relax it. Then watch your breathing-in and breathing-out. The breath must be deep, long and slow. You should fix your mind on inhale and exhale breaths with association of '*So-Ham*' or '*Ham-Sa*' mantra. Inhale with the mental sound of '*Ham*' and exhale with the mantle sound of '*Sa*' in a rhythm.

Next watch the thoughts in your mind. Thoughts may be coming in and going out. Your mind may be calm and peaceful. Just watch the thoughts coming in and going out as an un-interested film-observer. Do not indulge, struggle & attach yourself with your thoughts. *Concentrate on the Aggyia Chakra*, the point between the eyebrows. It is also known as *nasikagra* mentioned in Gita. *Nasikagra* is the point from where the nose starts, which is between the eyebrows. The other end of the nose is the end point and not the starting point *(nasikagra)*. It is a misconception among many yogis. They think just opposite.

When you deeply concentrate and are able to stop the incoming thoughts in your mind you will be blessed to see a light flame at Aggyia chakra. This is known as Third Eye of Shiva. Concentrate at this light. This light has not come from the outside world, but is the spark of the cosmic eternal light of God. It is in all of us. We all are in search of this. The thoughts inside all the men are always different, but this inner light of God is same in all. So, this is not an illusion or a myth, like the unwanted thoughts in your mind. This light is Truth, eternal, have no form, universal omnipresent and indestructible.

Try to go on concentrating inside this light, which is the source of ultimate knowledge of God. If any unwanted thought distracts your mind, try to ignore the thought. One day you will be blessed to see the special divine visions, which will unfold the secrets of the creation and weaken the bonds of *Maya*. A continuous meditation at this light will awaken the Kundalini inside you one day.

> *"The hearts of the people cry out the Lord...*
> *Let your tears flow like a river day and night...*
> *Arise; cry out in the night, Pour out your heart...*
> *Like water in the presence of the Lord."*
> **--- Lamentations 2:18-19**

Another Meditation Technique of Awakening Kundalini by a Kriya Yogi

The practice of this technique will liberate your soul imprisoned in the body from the bondages of five senses and the worldly things. It will enable your soul to merge with God or escape from your body through Sahasrara or any of the six chakras to unite with God at the time of death.

➤ *Practice*: Sit comfortably on your asana on a woolen blanket with your erect spine. Watch your whole body. If there is tension in any part of the body relax it. Watch your breath going in and going out. Make your breath deep and comfortable. Concentrate at Aggyia Chakra, the point between your eyebrows with slightly closed or half open eyes. Bring a smile and a peace on your face. Now slightly move your spine towards left and then towards right by swaying your body. Stop swaying the body after few seconds. Then try to move your inner consciousness up and down in your spine (Sushumana Nadi) from the Muladhara Chakra to Aggyia Chakra again and again. After that concentrate at the Muladhara Chakra and mentally chant the *Om* mantra. Continuing the chanting of *Om* mantra, shift your concentration at the Swadhisthan, Manipura, Anahata, Vishuddha and Aggyia Chakra one by one, gradually coming up the spine. Try to visualize and feel mentally the presence of the chakra with the number of petals described earlier at the right places in the spine, while chanting *Om* mantra repeatedly.

Similarly continue and repeat the same while going down from Aggyia Chakra to the Muladhara Chakra. Practice the same until you feel that your body consciousness has totally transferred from body into the spine. Try to remain awake and do not sleep during the practice. Very soon you will be lost in pure consciousness with bliss and joy.

Listening & Meditation on Anahata Sounds (Laya Yoga) or *Surat-Shabda* Yoga for a Kriya Yogi

It is the listening of the divine melody. In the beginning of creation of universe, God manifested Himself first in the form of "Word" (Om). *'Laya'* means dissolve or absorb. In Laya Yoga a state of mind is achieved, when one forgets all the objects of senses and gets absorbed in meditation. The practice of Laya enables one to have the perfect control over the five gross elements, mind and senses. The vibrant mind comes to rest. The body, mind and prana are subdued.

"It is said that mind is the lord of our senses, but breath is the lord of the mind and breath is slave of Anahat Nada."

For Laya Yoga, *Sambhavi Mudra* is an effective method, in which one intently concentrates on any one of the six Chakras. Trataka exercise plays a vital role in getting success in Laya yoga. Very soon, the yogi gets experience of Samadhi. He attains many Siddhis & liberation of soul.

Anahata sounds are the mystic sounds heard by the Yogis during deep meditation. Listening of the Anahat sounds is the sign of the purification of Nadis. The sound due to vibration of physical things does not produce these sounds. Yogi listen these sounds even if he closes his ears. Some aspirants hear these through only one ear, but some by both the ears. There are loud as well as feeble sounds. From the loud, one will have to contemplate on the feeble and from the feeble to the subtler. Beginners can hear the sound only when the ears are closed. Advanced yogis can concentrate on these Anahata sounds even without closing the ears. The ultimate Anahata sound is termed as *Omkara* (Om) sound. It is produced from the Anahata centre of the *Sushumana* Nadi.

➢ *Practice*: Sit comfortably in your usual Asana. Close the ears with the thumbs. Try to listen minutely and observe the internal sounds through the ears. When you hear these sounds from within you will not be able to listen the external sounds. Close your eyes. In the beginning of your practice, you will hear many loud sounds. Later the sounds are faded away. The mind is first forcibly concentrated on any one of the sounds out of many and fixed firmly to it till it is absorbed in it. The mind becomes one with the Anahat sound as the milk with water. Then it is rapidly absorbed in the mental space (*Chidakasa*). It is like the bee drinking the honey does not bother for anything else. Similarly, the mind, which is completely absorbed in the inner Anahat sound, cuts off its connection with all the sensual detaching objects.

The Anahata sound emanating from *Pranava* (Om) Nada is *Brahman*. It is of the nature of effulgence. The mind gets absorbed in it and this is known as the '*Turiya*' state of mind. It is the supreme state of consciousness. It is also known as the *Unmani* state. The body appears to be dead just as a log of wood and it stops feeling heat or cold, joy or sorrow.

There are of ten kinds of Anahat Nada. The first is like the sound '*Chini*'; the second is '*Chini-chini*'; the third is the sound of a *bell*; the fourth is that of a *conch*; the fifth is that of a *lute*; the sixth is the sound of *cymbals*; the seventh is the tune of a *flute*; the eighth is the voice of a *drum* (*Bheri*); the ninth is the sound of a *double-drum* (*Mridanga*); and the tenth is the sound of *thunder* (Om).

One cannot listen these sounds immediately after closing the ears. One should concentrate and keep the mind pin-pointed to listen the Anahat sounds. It is not necessary that a particular sound, which you have listened today, will also be listened every day. But you will always hear at least any one of the ten Anahata sounds.

As the yogi concentrates on Anahata sounds during meditation, similarly he should also meditate at the Aggyia chakra known as 'Third Eye', on any of the five gross elements, on *'So-ham'*, on *'Tat-tvam Asi'* and on *'Aham Brahma-Asmi'* the great statements of the Vedas.

Bhakti Yoga Technique[1]

Bhakti is the easiest and the simplest way of Kundalini awakening Kundalini. But it is a slow technique. One may take many births to achieve the ultimate aim. In Bhakti the aspirant should follow:-

- Listening, singing classical devotional songs or dancing in the glory of God, individually or with a group of disciples
- Attending Satsanga in the glory of God
- Visit and meditation at sacred religious places
- Complete surrender at the feet of God
- Simple living and following the Yama & Niyama
- Offerings and prayers to God
- Service of the humanity etc.

A Hatha Yogi achieves the highest stage of samadhi by the practice of various Mudras, Bandhas, Asanas, Pranayama and other exercises. A Raja-yogi or a Kriya-yogi achieves the same by deep concentration and meditation. A devotee

---

[1] For detail read Basis of Bhakti yoga in chapter 3rd

(*bhakta*) achieves by developing devotion & self-surrender to God. A *Jnana-yogi* achieves the same by the practice of *Sravana, Manana and Nididhyasana*. A *Karma-yogi* achieves by the selfless service to God and others. The final goal (communion with God) is the same in all the paths, but there are minute differences in their paths.

Raja-Yoga or Kriya-Yoga is the meditation on the different centers of energy (chakras). Jnana-Yoga is the concentration and meditation on the Kundalini Shakti. Hatha Yoga is the meditation at the different Chakras and Nadis and awakening the Kundalini Shakti through physical methods. Meditation on gods and the presiding deities of the Chakras is helpful for quick success. An aspirant may combine the different methods of yoga paths as per his individual ability and liking.

A devotee when meditates on the presiding deity, imagines the particular form of god at each Chakra. The Bhakta-yogi also gets various subtle visions and observes different forms of God.

Kriya Yoga Technique of Awakening Kundalini

There are some scriptural restrictions on Kriya Yoga technique. It is not revealed, unless one deserves it. After a long austere it will be more effective and beneficial. It will be still better if you get this technique directly through a self-realized guru. Through the 'intuitive eye' and tests a Guru knows, when to provide this technique to his disciple. The disciple also assures to be faithful to his Guru, his teachings and also practice the Kriya technique twice daily in the morning and evening. If one does not follow the rules of Kriya Yoga, one may not get as much benefit and may suffer due to improper awakening of the Kundalini.

For a Kriya yogi there is a day-to-day need of spiritual guidance of a Guru for further progress. For better benefit I will suggest you to become the member of the *God-Realization Foundation*[2]. It will provide you the detailed regular spiritual guidance as well as the e-Spiritual-Tests through its Internet services. It is most convenient and faster in the modern times.

The following is a brief description of techniques of Kriya-practice. A Guru passes on the details and a sacred mantra at the time of initiation. It requires sincerity to practice and dedication to Guru.

> Just before your Kriya it is always better to do Maha-Mudra as explained earlier.

> After your regular asanas, pranayams, exercises and bathing sit comfortable on your asana for meditation with erect spine. Watch, if there is any tension in any part of the body. Relax your whole body. Fix your concentration at Aggyia chakra.

> Watch your inhale and exhale breaths. Take a deep inhale breath with the inner sound of 'Ham' and exhale slowly with an inner sound of 'Sa'. Repeat for some time with a rhythm. This is breathing with 'So-Ham' or Ham-Sa mantra. 'So' means He and 'Ham' means I. 'So-Ham' means 'He is I'. Try to realize that you are one with He (God). It stops decay in body cells and organs. It calms the heart and the beats become slow.

---

[2] To become the member of GRF read the rules & regulations of 'God-Realization Foundation' page 231-2.

Your breathing will be dead slow. A Kriya yogi may practice the 'So-Ham' mantra throughout the day.

- Watch your thoughts. Your mind should be at rest without any unwanted thoughts. Concentrate at Aggyia chakra. Chant repeatedly the long Pranava-Mantra 'Aum' as many times as you can, so that your mind is totally merged in it. Try to listen the inner Cosmic Anahat Sound of Aum and concentrate on it. One has to meditate on Aum Sound to contact with God. After this, mentally chant Aum, Aum, Aum.... for some time without movement of tongue and any sound. Concentrate on any Anahat sound you listen.

- A Kriya yogi should first mentally directs the life-force (*prana*) to move it upward and downward through his Sushumana nadi, piercing the six chakras in the spine.

- Take a deep and slow inhaling breath through your mouth. While inhaling try to force the life energy to move upward from the Muladhara to Aggyia chakra along with a feeble inner sound of 'Ahhh...'

- Rest for a while; exhale through your open mouth slowly. Try to force the life-energy to flow downward, from Aggyia chakra to Muladhara with a feeble sound of 'Eeee...'. The sounds of 'Ahhh...' & 'Eeee...' should not be audible externally. These are chanted mentally only.

- Try to feel the sensation of coolness in your Sushumana nadi while you inhale and try to feel the sensation of warmness in Sushumana nadi while you exhale. While inhaling feel a cool current is flowing upward and while

Techniques of Awakening The Kundalini

exhaling feel a hot current is flowing downward inside Sushumana nadi. This is one cycle of breath.

> Intermix the *prana* with *apana* currents and apana with prana current while inhaling and exhaling. Retain your breath for a short while after inhalation and then exhale slowly. After exhalation wait for a moment for next inhale. The whole cycle of breathing should be done slowly and peacefully with a rhythm, without any strain and unwanted thoughts. This is known as one *Kriya*.

> A perfect Kriya cycle takes nearly 30 seconds duration. In the beginning, a Kriya Yogi is allowed to perform 14 Kriyas in one sitting, twice daily in morning and evening. Later it can be increased to 24 or 48 with the permission of the Guru.

> During the practice it is important that a Kriya yogi mentally directs the prana energy to flow upward and downward, piercing about the six centers of chakras (whirlpool of pranic energy) in the spinal cord. These six centers of chakras correspond to the twelve astral zodiacal signs (*Rashies*) also known as the Cosmic Man.

> After the Kriya practice one should do the Jyoti Mudra as described earlier. During the Meditation or Jyoti Mudra one may be blessed to see the 'Third Eye' or the 'Spiritual Eye' at the Aggyia chakra or he may listen the Anahat sound of Aum. The spiritual eye is the mystic door to God revelation. The light of God illuminates the entire cosmic consciousness. It generally of golden color. Within this light a dark blue color ball of light is visible. It is profoundly serene. Within this blue sphere a five-pointed bright white star

is visible. Try to concentrate and penetrate this five-pointed star with the japa of 'Om, Om, Om...'. It is the door to God-realization. If yogi is able to listen the Anahat sound of Aum, then he should meditate on it (read Laya yoga).

Whatever is in the macrocosm is also in the microcosm. The inner and outer universes are identical and inter-liked with each other. These affect Kriya yogi in a practice of half minute Kriya. The spinal cord is apparently magnetized. The flow of up-down prana energy around the six sensitive chakras in spine increases the normal (slow) evolution of human life tremendously. *The evolution of man in a half minute of Kriya practice is equivalent to the normal (slow) evolution of one year. This creates a significant difference in the human spiritual evolution.*

Occasionally, when the prana is absorbed in the spiritual eye an advanced Kriya yogi may experience breathlessness or samadhi or Kundalini awakening. The technique relaxes the body, mind and the nervous system. It decarbonizes the blood and over-charges it with oxygen. The oxygen is transmuted into prana and is directed to flow into Sushumana penetrating the chakras. The absolute truth is revealed.

!Om Anandam Om!

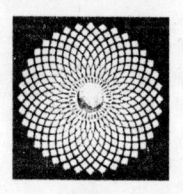

8

Experiences After Awakening Kundalini

Prayer

Experiences Before & After Awakening The Kundalini

The Symptoms of Awakening the Kundalini

Flow of Life Currents After Awakening the Kundalini

How an Aspirant should Live After Awakening of Kundalini

Misconceptions of Awakening of Kundalini

Eight Major Siddhis After Awakening

Many Minor Siddhis (Riddhis)

Experiences and Symptoms of Awakening of Kundalini

General Precautions to be taken care off after Awakening of the Kundalini

What Happens when Kundalini pierces:
Muladhara, Swadhisthan, Manipur, Anahata, Vishuddha and Aggyia Chakras

What happens when the Kundalini pierces the Sahasrara?

The Problems of Improper Awakening of Kundalini

Does Awakening of Kundalini Means Self-Realization or the Enlightenment?

8

8
Experiences After
Awakening the Kundalini

Prayer

O Mother Divine! O Mystic Creative Cosmic Power! What an extraordinary mystic game Thou art playing with Thy children? Thou art the Vehicle of the soul for involution in the journey back to God. Thou art the destroyer of Illusion, Delusion, *Maya*[1] and Ignorance. Thou art the Divine Pure Love to unite with God.

O Mother of All! Through Thy infinite grace and power, dissolve our mind, illumines our intellect and make us realize our original identity with the Supreme Brahman, Father of All. May Thy Blessings be upon all!

---

[1] For details of Illusion, Delusion & Maya read the chapter 1 of the book God & Self-Realization (Scientific & Spiritual View) by Sh. Dharam Vir Mangla.

Experiences Before and After Awakening of The Kundalini

An aspirant may experience some strange mystic behaviors and internal personality crisis, even before the awakening of the Kundalini. There may be the series of disappointments, a feeling of guilt, a growing sense of dissatisfaction, a moral crisis, a change in personal interests and feeling of something missing. There are significant variations in the experiences, depending upon the fruits of past karmas and the *yog-sadhana* (yoga-practice) of the aspirants. These change in behaviors are the remarkable symptoms of the progress of spiritual achievement of an aspirant. He should not be afraid of these changes.

When Kundalini is sleeping and dormant, man is awakened to the outer world. But when it awakes, the man sleeps to the outer world. He looses his interests and consciousness of the world and enters into his causal body. The awakening of the Kundalini is the culmination of a series of prayers, meditation practices, penances and austerities as prescribed in all the major religions. Through the regular practices & efforts, the aspirant receives the divine grace of God and Guru to awaken his Kundalini.

Many times the awakening of Kundalini is a blissful extraordinary spiritual experience. It is powerful like the blast of a rocket lunching. So the aspirant should avoid, the forceful arousing of Kundalini without purification of his body, mind and basic knowledge of the mystic Kundalini yoga and proper guidance.

In many cases it is possible that the activeness of the Kundalini energy may be extremely subtle and unnoticeable. The aspirant may not be aware of the awakening of his Kundalini at all. On the other hand so many *Sadhaks* (aspirants) wrongly presume that their Kundalini has awakened. It leads to their false pride of achievement.

As soon as Kundalini is awakened, it pierces the Muladhara chakra. The yogi should try to lift it to the Sahasrara through the Sushumana Nadi. When Kundalini pierces a chakra, an intense heat is felt there. When it leaves the chakra, it becomes cold and lifeless. The aspirant achieves so many siddhies when Kundalini pierces a chakra. He gets the victory over the five gross elements one by one. When it reaches *Sahasrara*, the yogi experiences the *Chida-akasa* (ocean/ space of knowledge). Remember, it is easier to awaken the Kundalini but difficult to raise it to the Sahasrara. As Kundalini proceeds to higher centers of energy, divine Knowledge is received intuitively,

Some times a sudden contact with the subtle truths and reality is incomprehensible to understand by the aspirant. The absolute reality & truth is unknown to worldly people. Many times this leads to some psychic disorders and adjustment with the world. But the aspirant should carefully adjust himself with his family, friends, society and the world and should not become nervous.

The Symptoms of Awakening the Kundalini

If the aspirant experiences any or some of the following symptoms, it may be due to the awakening of his Kundalini. Then he must be very careful about it.

➢ Frequent feeling or sensation of hot or ice-cold currents flowing up and down in the spinal region.

- A tingling feeling in the spine, abdomen and the head.
- Body restlessness and vibrations in the arms, legs, palms and feet.
- The pulse rate and alertness are increased. Blood pressure is reduced.
- Cholesterol, fat and acid level in the body are reduced. Cardiac and brain waves are stabilized. The irregular growth and formation of cancer cells are retarded.
- A feeling of something like snake wriggling up in the spine from the *Muladhara* chakra to *Vishuddha* chakra.
- The aspirant becomes sensitive to the *Anahat* sounds, noise, bright lights and strong smells.
- There are various visions of cosmic world and mystic experiences. The aspirants are gifted with the revelation of cosmic secrets and achieve many *Riddhis and Siddhis*.
- Sometimes sleeplessness and mental depression comes. The aspirant should try to keep him away from crowd and live aloof.
- There may be frequent emotional disturbance and outbursts like: changes in mood, unknown fear, grief, depression, sudden laughing, uncontrolled crying and hiccups etc.
- Hearing of the Anahat (inner) sounds (Voice of God) like that of *damroo (musical instrument in the hand of Shiva)*, flute, rain, drum, waterfall, chirping birds, buzzing, whooshing, ringing bells and ringing even if the ears are closed. These Anahat sounds have a soothing, comforting and protecting effect.
- There are various visions of inner subtle Lights of God. The aspirant is connected with God through these inner lights and sounds. The inner Light is of many colors. A blue colored solid sphere surrounded by a golden hollow sphere, with a five-pointed white star at the center is also visible. It is generally known as '*Third*

Eye'. If the aspirant has not followed the true path of yoga, the inner Light may blind him for several days. Sri Sidheshwar Baba (Dr. B. S Goel, Founder of Third eye Mission) encountered strong inner lights of many colors with his closed eyes. Lights were so strong that he could not sleep for several days due to the fear of the closing the eyes.

- The aspirant automatically gets the victory over the five enemies: *Kama* (sex), *Krodha* (anger), *Mad* (pride), *Lobh* (passion) and *Moha* (attachment).
- The freedom from worldly desires is achieved.
- A deep peace of mind is attained beyond description.
- Yogi feels a compassion and love for all. He feels grateful even to his critics and enemies.
- The sex instinct is automatically controlled and balanced. The aspirant feels that he is neither a body nor a male nor a female.
- Yogi achieves pure state of intellectual wisdom and power to transcend him to merge in Supreme God.
- Some of the aspirants are gifted to choose the mode, place and time of their death (*Mahasamadhi*) as per their will. Many of the great yogis like Sri Paramhansa Yogananda, his Gurus: Yukteshwar Giri and Lahari Mahashyia and numerous other saints took their Mahasamadhis (leaving the physical body) at their sweet will. They all predicted their mode, place and time in advance.

A Yoga aspirant should know the symptoms of the awakening of the *Kundalini Shakti,* since his Kundalini may awaken any day. If the yogi doesn't know these symptoms, then he will be afraid of the abnormal subtle things, which he may likely going to experience. No doctor or family members or worldly persons will be able to understand his extraordinary symptoms and problems. He may wrongly presume that some mysterious power like a ghost or a devil has overpowered him. Many times an aspirant may falsely presume that his Kundalini has awakened.

During the awakening of the Kundalini, an aspirant may be blessed to experience the smell of many mystic perfumes; tastes of mystic things, divine feelings of touch, divine visions of mystic worlds and the *Anahat* sounds. His *Viveka* (intuitive power) may increase significantly. Aspirant may receives the knowledge about the past & future direct from the God. There may be some sensation or pulsation in the *Muladhara chakra*. His hairs of the body may erect at their roots and the aspirant enjoys a state of bliss and Ananda. His breathing may stop for a short duration, all of a sudden (*Kevala Kumbhak),* but without any discomfort or exertion.

The aspirant should not fear & worry about these. He should realize that his *Kundalini* is now active & awakened. But now he must be very careful to follow all the *Yama* and *Niyama* as per the scriptures and not as some of the authors misinterpret. Mother Kundalini does not tolerate the violation of *Yama* and *Niyama* by the aspirant. No aspirant can escape from the omni watching eyes of Kundalini.

During his meditation the yogi gets intuition power (*viveka*), insights and inspirations of subtle things. The Mother Nature unfolds the secrets of creation one by one and all the doubts are cleared. Vedas are realized within without reading actually and their meaning becomes self-evident. Clearly it is symptom of activation and awakening of the Kundalini.

If the *aspirant does the Uddiyana, Jalandhara and Mulabandha involuntarily*, it is also a clear symptom of awakening of *Kundalini* and its activation. The aspirant sometimes feels the vibrations of strong prana (life force) rising up in the spinal cord towards Sahasrara in different parts of his body. Sometimes the aspirant experiences the electric shocks in his body specially the spine. He begins to perform the asanas *involuntarily* without any pain and difficulty.

Some times the aspirant repeats the mantras involuntarily. Aspirant achieves the state of thoughtlessness with awareness, for a long time. He is surprised to experience that he is not a physical body. His eyes are closed automatically. He is not able to open his eyes inspite of his best efforts. It is also a clear symptom of his *Kundalini* is active.

Some times the body of aspirant becomes weightless and light. He is able to fly in air easily. Aspirant gets inexhaustible energy to work continuously for hours, without any fatigue, sleep or food. He begins to understand the clear meaning of his dreams. His memory becomes very sharp. His intelligence is increased significantly. He may be blessed to compose magnificent hymens and poetry, like saints Tulsi Das, Meera, Kabeer and Guru Nanak.

Flow of Life Currents After Awakening the Kundalini

After the awakening, the dormant static potential Kundalini power becomes a dynamic. The life current begins to move through the coiled passage at the coccygeal region from the downward-bent lotus chakras to upward towards brain.

Initially the petals of lotuses inside the chakras and these are bent downward.

But when the Kundalini crosses the chakras, the petals of lotuses are turned upward. The petals emit the rays of different wavelengths and connect these life-currents with the concerned nerves, which further perform the various functions in the body. The reverse life current flows through the coiled coccyx towards the brain. Then the ego 'I' disconnects its association with the physical body, five senses and sex organs.

We know the vibrations of radio, TV or mobile phones etc. are unheard, undetected and unseen without the help of a proper scientific instrument like radio, TV or mobile phone. These vibrations pass silently without our knowledge and observation. Similarly there are many other vibrations of the finer subtle forces and the subtle voices of angles and gods. These are present in *ether* and are passing through the cosmic vibration unheard, unseen and un-noticed by us. The awakening of Kundalini converts our brain into like a spiritual radio or TV or mobile phone receiver to enables us to observe and listen the music of these vibrations.

The awakening of Kundalini disconnects the five sensory motor telephones (senses) from the body. It enables the life energy to accumulate in the brain. Then it is connected to an ocean of Knowledge (Chit-Akasha), like a grand spiritual TV channel. Then our brain receives the unheard music of the electrons, atomic particles, the finer electromagnetic waves and the cosmic vibratory voice of God. All the life forces, all the atomic particles, all the electromagnetic waves and all the cosmic vibrations have their special music sounds. But the human ear is unable to hear these music sounds. After awakening of Kundalini, the aspirant is able to make celestial connections and listen these music sounds of God's creation.

How an Aspirant should live After the Awakening of Kundalini

- The aspirant should follow strictly all the *Yama & Niyama* as per the scriptures and not as per some of the ignorant authors.
- Take proper guidance from a self-realized Guru*.
- Meditate more (for hours); attend Satsanga (spiritual songs & lectures by saints).
- Do asanas, pranayama and exercises regularly.
- Chant Om and the mantra given by your Guru with full concentration at the Aggyia Chakra for many minutes and many times a day.
- Keep *Mauna* (silence) for the maximum time and avoid useless talk and discussions.
- Frequent bathing and wearing simple clean cloths is useful.
- Avoid frequent contact with worldly people with negative thoughts. Try to remain away from crowds. But not a group *Satsanga*.
- Avoid sexual life for some time. Control the sexual instincts and desires. Extra marital sex is strictly prohibited. One cannot befool Kundalini Shakti.
- In case of physical bodily problems due to Kundalini, the doctors will not be of much help. Avoid taking medicines, drugs, smoking, alcohol and non-vegetarian food.

---

*To understand better, who is a self-realized Guru, read the book "God & Self-Realization" (Scientific & Spiritual View) by Sh. Dharam Vir Mangla.

- Take only the *satwik* food, plenty of milk, fruits, vegetables, almonds, small-cardamom and observe fruit or juice fast frequently. The cold lemon-juice with sugar, water and salt is very useful.
- Read the Scriptures like Bhagwad Geeta and good spiritual books daily.
- The members of your family will not be able to understand your inner mystic spiritual experiences and abnormal behavior. They may be unnecessarily worried and confused about you. Try to convince them that nothing is wrong with you, and you need not seek the help of any doctor. You will be all right after some time.
- A Pranic or a Reiki healing therapy may be helpful in controlling the problems related with awakening.
- Sometimes the further spiritual progress is stopped and aspirant gets discouraged. In such times consult your Guru and meditate more.

Misconceptions of Awakening of Kundalini by Many Authors

In most of the ordinary worldly persons life force is moving downward through coiled the passage and stimulates the sex organs of both in male and female. By the constant efforts, will power & celibacy an aspirant reverses the flow upwards. Even the most powerful microscope or any physical instrument can't detect the flow of the life energy in the body downward or upward in the spine.

Some of the western Authors and Tantriks are now apparently busy these days in interpreting and translating the Holy Hindu Scriptures from Sanskrit to other languages. Although they are doing a great work, but they are writing the spiritual topics about which they don't have much knowledge. Most of them have been brought up and grown up in a modern western culture and environment, which generally lacks moral ethics of sex and does not concern with the spirituality and God. They neither have done their spiritual *sadhana* (yoga practice), nor they got an opportunity or guidance from the self-realized Gurus, nor they got the opportunity of the company of saints and sages, nor do they understand the difference between an Avatara or a Guru or a saint or a Sanyasi or an ordinary spiritual teacher. They do not understand clearly most of the yogic-terms.

Due to their insufficient little learning about the Hindu Scriptures, they are likely to misunderstand and misinterpret them. Due to their false imagination, ignorance and ill-logic they are misinterpreting Scriptures in their own ways. According to some of them Kundalini is an actual physical coiled sleeping serpent, residing and hidden at the base of the spine embedded within the vertebrae. They even presume that the awakened serpent Kundalini may bite the man and it may cause death to an aspirant. Some presume that the Kundalini is a sex force in men. This is due to their over-indulgence in sex instincts, and they can't even think of the control of their sex instinct and celibacy, which is necessary for the aspirant. For them sex and morality have no value. Morality lies in the power of resistance of evil. They cleverly twist the truth, *Yama & Niyama* to please their readers.

There is a recent instance of one self-declared God-man having millions of his following all over the world. He had no faith in the existence of God. He deliberately criticized and discarded the most of the religions, their ethical & moral values, and legal sex between the married couples. He was against the sacred marriage system of all the religions and mischievously justified the freely open immoral unethical combined group-sex among thousands of men and women with anybody like the animals. It is true that most of the people do not like celibacy and other moral ethics of Yama & Niyama imposed upon them by the Scriptures. Naturally they are attracted to a person, who justifies their immorality, as morality and religious too. Beware of such fake God-men. For increasing the number of their disciples, they may twist, sacrifice and manipulate the Scriptures to any extent.

Such authors are very susceptible to sex and immoral thoughts. They have taken only the elementary lessons on unscientific meditations from here and there. But due to their strong over-sex indulgence, they are unable to think other then sex during their unscientific meditation. During the meditation, their mind simply roams in the ocean of sex and the powerful crocodile-of-sex overpowers them.

They may feel exiting sensations in their sex regions and falsely claim, presume and declare that their Kundalini has awakened. They approach to their inner-guide counselor, who advises them to stop further meditation and misinform them that their Kundalini has awakened. In fact the inner-guide counselor himself has no experience of awakening of the Kundalini. To call Kundalini power as sex force is nothing but a short of intentional mischief. For a man of intemperance or dissipation it is most difficult to awaken the Kundalini.

Some authors misadvise their aspirants to presume themselves as Lord Shiva and all the ladies as Ma Shakti. They falsely presume that the sexual union is the easiest and best way of merging of Lord Shiva with Ma Shakti. Some begins to worship their spouses too, with lustful propensities. All such practices lead the aspirants nowhere.

The drinking of the nectar or divine intoxication or ecstasy mentioned in the Scriptures has been mostly misinterpreted by them, as the drinking of wine, drugs and other intoxicants. The aspirants, who believe on them, simply waste their life in fool's paradise and become self-deluded souls.

The sex instinct can be controlled easily by the mystic spiritual experiences during meditation, but one has to control his sex thoughts during meditation. As only the light can destroy the darkness, similarly the correct meditation as mentioned in the scriptures can definitely help in the victory over the strong sex thoughts. Believe that only after the sex is conquered the Kundalini can be awakened.

From the above, do not conclude that the sex is completely prohibited for an aspirant and one has to leave his spouse and family to observe celibacy. But one must be moderate in sex with his legal spouse. The immoral sex with others and with anybody is strictly prohibited for a yogi. We cannot befool God, from his omniwatching eyes. God has not deprived the family holders from awakening their Kundalini, but one must observe the *Yama & Niyama* as defined in the Scriptures. Most of the great self-realized saints (*Rishies*) have been the family-holders in the past and some were even the kings.

Sri Gopi Krishna has written in his book 'Kundalini Yoga': "Real food for nervous system is bio-plasma, an essence from sex glands which ascends via spinal cord upto the brain". The celibacy is most useful in the awakening and rising up the Kundalini.

I strongly disagree with the views of Swami Satyananda Saraswati, Dr. Ravinder Kumar and many other authors about their opinion that the aspirants who observe *Brahmacharya* (celibacy and remain bachelor for whole life) are likely to suffer terrible headaches on awakening of the Kundalini. The following conclusion is most illogical, unfortunate, without any statistics and a misleading statement from Swami Satyananda Saraswati, as stated in his book:

"Some aspirants experience terrible headaches when Kundalini is awakening, however this does not mean that all headaches are related to Kundalini and not everybody will have headaches. Generally, <u>those who have had married life do not have this experience. It is usually only those who have not had any kind of sexual interactions who experience headaches with the advent of Kundalini awakening.</u>"

It is remarkable that Siddheswar Baba (Dr. B.S. Goel), the author of "Third Eye and Kundalini" and other books, suffered a sever headache on his awakening of the Kundalini. But it is absolutely illogical and wrong to write by Dr. Ravinder Kumar in his book "Kundalini for Beginners" that the cause of his terrible headache was: "He (Dr. B.S. Goel) remained unmarried for the whole life". He should know that there had been thousands of examples of no-headaches by the whole life bachelor and celibate aspirants, who suffered no-headaches on awakening of their Kundalini and there had been so many married couples, who suffered lot of problems including the headaches on awakening of their Kundalini.

You must be convinced that a regulated balanced sex life is a must between the married partner aspirants. Still a bachelor and a celibacy-married life are far better to awaken the Kundalini without any problems.

Eight Major *Siddhis*

By the awakening of the mystic power of Kundalini a yogi achieves some of the eight major *Siddhis*, viz., *Anima, Mahima, Laghima, Garima, Prapti, Prakamya, Vasitvam* and *Ishitvam*.

1. ***Anima Siddhi***: An aspirant is able to diminish his physical body as minute as he pleases, e.g. Hanuman.

2. ***Mahima Siddhi***: *Mahima* is the opposite of Anima. Aspirant can enlarge his body as big as he likes. The whole universe can be inside him, e.g. Hanuman & Kumbhkaran.

3. ***Laghima Siddhi***: Aspirant can make his body as light as air. He can levitate and lift his body suspended in the air. His body floats easily in air and he can walk on water too. The body can be made light by *Plavini* pranayama. Some of the yogi can travel with speed close to light in the sky with the help of this *Siddhi*, e.g. Hanuman & *Rakshasas* like Ravana, Meghanad (son of Ravana) and many others.

4. ***Garima Siddhi***: This is the opposite of Laghima. By this Siddhi the yogi can make his body as heavy as he likes, like a mountain with high huge gravity, e.g. Angad the son of Bali in Ramayana.

5. ***Prapti Siddhi***: The yogi is able to touch the Sun or the Moon or the sky. The yogi is able to attain all his desires. He gets supernatural powers like the clairvoyance, the power of predicting future events, clairaudience, telepathy and thought reading of others etc. He can understand any unknown language including the language of the beasts and birds. He achieves the super power to cure diseases of

others, e.g. Bhagavan Ved-Vyas, Hanuman, Sri Sathya Sai Baba and Mahavtar Babaji etc.

6. *Prakamya Siddhi*: Aspirant is able to live inside water for as much time as he desires. The late Tralinga Swami of Varanasi[*] used to live continuously for months underneath the Ganges. Yogi also gets the power to make his body invisible or visible as per his will (Mahavtar Baba Ji[*]). Yogi gets the power to enter the body of someone else. Sri Adi Shankarcharaya[*] entered the body of Raja Amaruka of Varanasi. Tirumular a saint of Southern India entered the body of a shepherd. Raja Vikramaditya also had this power. Yogi gets the power of keeping his youth appearance for any length of time. Raja Yayati also had this power.

7. *Vasitvam Siddhi*: It is the power of taming wild animals and bringing them under one's control. It is the power of mesmerizing and strong will to make the persons and living creatures obedient e.g. King Bharata, Lord Rama & Lord Krishna etc.

8. *Ishitvam Siddhi*: By the attainment of this divine siddhi a yogi becomes like the lord of the universe. A yogi with this siddhi can give life even to dead. Sri Satya Sai Baba, Jesus Christ, Ved-Vyas, Mahavtar Babaji and so many others has this power of bringing back life to the dead.

---

[*] To know about Tralinga Swami, Adi Shankarcharaya & Mahavtar Baba Ji, Sri Satya Sai Baba and so many saints, consult the book "God & Self-Realization (Scientific & Spiritual View)" by Sh. Dharam Vir Mangla.

The Minor *Siddhis* (*Riddhis*)

A yogi may acquires the following minor *Siddhis* known as *Riddhis* on awakening the Kundalini Shakti:

1. Freedom from the effects of heat and cold e.g. Sri Tralinga Swami and so many.

2. Freedom from *Raga-Dvesha* e.g. Sri Sathya Sai Baba & Mahavtar Babaji.

3. Clairvoyance (Vision of far places) i.e. *Doora-Darshan* like Tele-Vision e.g. Sri Ved-Vyas and Sanjay of Mahabharata and Nostradamus etc.

4. Clairaudience (Listen from far places) i.e. *Doora-Sravan / Sruti / Pravachana* e.g. Sri Ved-Vyas, Sanjay and Nostradamus etc.

5. *Mano-Jaya* (Victory over Mind) e.g. Mahavtar Babaji & Sri Satya Sai Baba etc.

6. The Yogi can take any form he likes i.e. *Kama Rupa* e.g. Ravana, Mareech, Hanuman etc.

7. *Parakaya Pravesha*: Yogi can enter into the body of another man. He can also animate a dead body and enter into it by transferring his soul e.g. Adi Shankaracharaya.

8. *Iccha-Mrityu*: Yogi gets the victory over his death & can die at his will e.g. Bhism Pitamaha, Mahavtar Babaji, Paramhansa Yogananda and Shirdi Sai Baba.

9. *Devanam Saha Kreeda* and *Darshana*: Yogi gets the vision and plays with deities e.g. Lahari Mahashyia, Lord Krishna.

10. *Yatha Sankalpa*: Yogi gets whatever he wishes and likes e.g. Sri Sathya Sai Baba.

11. *Trikala-Jnana*: Knowledge of past, present and future e.g. Mahavatar Babaji and Sri Sathya Sai Baba.

12. *Advandva*: Beyond the pairs of opposites. So many achieve this.

13. *Vak-Siddhi*: Whatever the Yogi predicts will happen i.e. true prophecy, e.g. Most of the gods & spiritual men (Rishies) of Sat-yuga & Treta-yuga had this power.

14. The Yogi can turn any metal into gold & gold into metal or sand or anything. So many yogis can do it.

15. *Kaya-Vyuha*: Yogi can manifest as many body as he likes to exhaust his Karmas in one life e.g. Mahavtar Babaji, Swami Pranavananda etc.

16. *Darduri-Siddhi*: The jumping power like a frog.

17. *Patala-Siddhi*: Yogi achieves victory over all the desires, destroys sorrows and diseases. So many achieve this.

18. Yogi gets the knowledge of his past lives e.g. *Bhisma* Pitamaha, Lord Krishna & many others.

19. Yogi gets knowledge of the cluster of stars and planets e.g. Maharishi Bhirgu.

20. Yogi gets the power of perceiving & contacting the *Siddhas* and gods in the astral worlds e.g. Lahari Mahashyia

Experiences After Awakening the Kundalini

21. Yogi gets mastery over the five gross elements: Earth, Water, Fire, Air, Ether and, mastery over the Prana. Almost all gets this power.
22. *Kama-chari*: One can move to any place he likes. Sri Narada, Adi Shankaracharaya, Mahavtar Babaji and Amar Jyoti Babaji.
23. Yogi gets the power of omnipotence, omnipresence and omniscience.
24. Yogi is able to point out the underground places, where a hidden treasure lies.
25. Freedom from hunger and thirst e.g. Giri Bala, Tralinga Swami, Mahavtar Babaji and so many.
26. *Vayu-Siddhi*: Yogi becomes light, levitate and rises in the air above the ground and remain suspended as long as he likes. So many get it including the *Rakshasas*.

General Precautions to be taken care off After Awakening the Kundalini

➢ But if the yogi is not able to pierce his Swadhisthan chakra to cross the Kundalini upward, he will be holding back his earthly energies like passions, sexual aggressions & infatuations etc.
➢ During the period of awakening of the Kundalini a disciple should remain in contact with his Guru or Spiritual Master, who has already awakened his own Kundalini and is self-realized also.
➢ If the Kundalini starts moving up through the Ida or Pingla Nadis instead of Sushumana, then the aspirant may be in trouble. If it moves through Ida (cool), he may suffer from kidney failure or stones in gall bladder or liver problems etc. If Kundalini moves through

Pingla (hot), he may suffer from over-sex instinct and become lusty.
> If the aspirant is not able the cross the chakras, he may become depressed, nervous, suspicious and of unstable mood. One should avoid opening the chakras forcibly as the chakras may be damaged.

All the chakras have a number of nadis emanating from each of the petal of the chakra lotus. Each petal has a special music sound of some syllable of Sanskrit language. When the Kundalini is dormant the syllables work mechanically. But when it is awakened, the syllables emit energy within them.

What Happens when Kundalini Pierces: The Muladhara Chakra

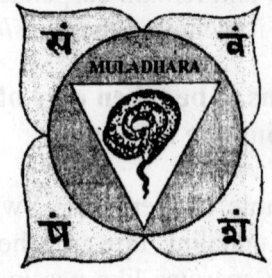

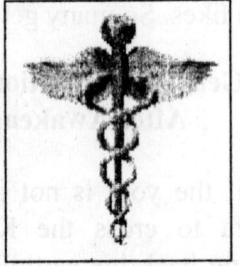

Muladhara Chakra   Kundalini Rising

Description of Muladhara Chakra as observed by the Aspirant

Shape	Four petalled Lotus
Size	8 cm x 8 cm. Rotates clockwise
Location Male	Below the Testis
Female	Near the mouth of Uterus
Nadis	Vam, Sham, Scham, Sam
Bija Mantra	Lam

Granthi	Brahma Granthi
Loka	Bhu Loka
Color of Nadis	Deep Red
Vayu	Apana
Yantra	Square
Element/Color	Earth / Yellow
Goddess	Dakini / Savitri
God	Ganesha
God Element	Mahakal Sharpa (Coiled snake)
God Energy	Lingam
Cont. Planet	Mars
Control. Deity	Indra
Animal	Aravat Elephant
Energy Centre	Yoni (Inverted Triangle)
Related Other Minor Chakras	*Eight*. Rudra-Charchika, Rudra-Chamunda, Siddh-Chamunda, Siddh-Laxmi, Siddh-Yogeshwari, Roop-Vidya, Shyama & Dhantura.

What Happens When Muladhara Chakra is opened

- The aspirant gets his victory over the gross earth (solids) elements.
- A tingling warm or cold sensation is felt in the spine at frequent intervals. Sometimes a high voltage lightening current is felt going up from Muladhara to Sahasrara.
- The aspirant gets the experience of his astral body. His body becomes light and weightless. He can levitate during meditation. He is able to come out and return to his physical body at his will during the meditation.
- The yogi is able to detach his etheric body from his physical. The detachment helps in the expansion of the body.

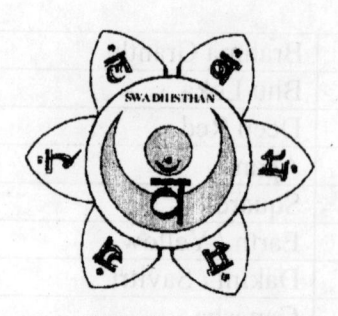

Swadhisthan Chakra
Description of Swadhisthan Chakra as observed

Shape	Six petalled Lotus
Location	Coccyx. Lowest end of spine.
Nadis	Six. Bam, Bham, Mam, Yam, Ram, Lam
Bija Mantra	Vam
Granthi	Brahma Granthi
Loka	Bhuvar Loka
Color of Nadis	Vermilion
Vayu	Vyana
Yantra	Crescent Moon
Element/Color	Water / White
Goddess	Rakini / Saraswati
God	Vishnu
God Element	Seshnag (Thousand headed snake)
God Energy	Crescent Moon
Control. Deity	Lord Vishnu
Animal	Crocodile
Energy Centre	Penis in male & Ovary in Female
Related Other Minor Chakras	*Ten.* Tarala, Ramani, Tarani, Bhanavi, Naini, Jainti, Indarani-Asthibakshi, Agneyi-Mamsapriya, Yama-Mahadamstra and Nairutti-Dirghadamstra.

What Happens When Swadhisthan Chakra is opened

- The yogi gets victory over the water (all fluids) element. He looses his fears due to water and fluids.
- The yogi is able to taste any thing he likes.
- The aspirant becomes very sensitive.
- Secret astral energies are revealed to the yogi.
- The aspirant gets the knowledge of his past, present and future lives.
- The aspirant experiences a buoyant force on his body, which makes his body light and float in the air.
- His sixth sense of the intuitive power is increased.
- Anahat sound of waves of water is felt at the Swadhisthan chakra.
- If the yogi is unable to open the Manipur chakra, then the Kundalini falls back to Muladhara chakra. He should try again & again to pierce Manipur chakra to move upwards.

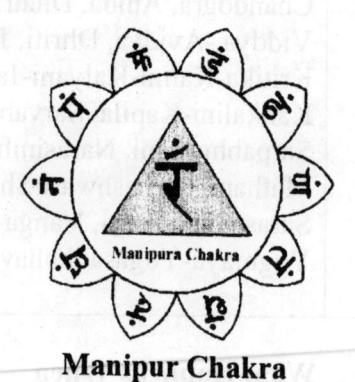

Manipur Chakra

Description of Manipur Chakra as observed by the Aspirant

Shape	Ten petalled Lotus
Location	Behind Navel

Nadis	Ten: Dam, Dham, Nam, Tam, Tham, Dam, Dham, Nam, Pam, Fam
Bija Mantra	Ram
Granthi	Brahma Granthi
Loka	Swarg or Svah Loka
Color of Nadis	Blue
Vayu	Samana
Yantra	Triangle
Element/Color	Fire (Agni) / Red
Goddess	Laxmi / Lakini
God	Rudra
God Element	Fire Triangle
God Energy	Fire
Control. Deity	Fire
Animal	Ram
Energy Centre	Navel
Related Other Minor Chakras	Twenty-two. Adya, Bhima, Brahma-Manya, Ajita, Brahavadini, Chandika, Chandogra, Amba, Dhatri, Agnihotri, Viddya,-Avidya, Dhriti, Jayavijaya-Jaya, Kritika-Kalini-Kalyani-Jalodhari, Kankalini-Kapila, Sarvabhutadamani-Sarpabhushani, Narasimhi, Madanon-Mathani, Maheshwari-Shankarpriya, Saraswati-Savitri, Vanga-Virupa and Yogmaya-Yogasadhbhava-Yogini.

What Happens When Manipur Chakra is opened?

➢ The aspirant gets victory over the gross Fire element and all kind of his fears and phobias. He begins to worship Fire as god.
➢ His digestive system is improved and stomach becomes free from diseases.

- Many riddhis (minor Siddhis) are achieved.
- A tremendous flow of energy begins to flow like a flooded river in the spine.
- His own body becomes free from diseases and he is able to understand the actual cause of problem of the diseases of other persons.
- The yogi gets the power to concentrate the vital energies inside higher unopened chakras.

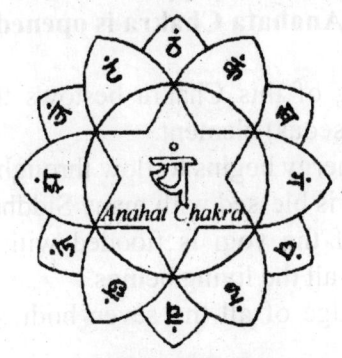

Anahata Chakra

Description of Anahat Chakra as observed by Aspirant

Shape	Twelve petalled Lotus
Location	Behind Heart
Nadis	Twelve. Kam, Kham, Gam, Gham, Dam, Cham, Chham, Jam, Jham, Nyam, Tam and Tham
Bija Mantra	Yam
Granthi	Vishnu Granthi
Loka	Mahar Loka
Color of Nadis	Red
Vayu	Prana
Yantra	Hexagonal (six pointed star)
Element/ color	Air / smoky
Goddess	Maha-Kali / Kakini

God	Ishana Rudra, Shankar
God Element	Triangle
God Energy	Air
Control. Deity	Air
Animal	Antelope
Energy Centre	Heart

What Happens When Anahata Chakra is opened

- The opening of this Chakra bestows the victory over gross air (gaseous) element.
- Kundalini energy begins to flow throughout the body.
- The aspirant is blessed with many Siddhis.
- The heart of the yogi is flooded with divine love & affection for all the living beings.
- The knowledge of all the seven bodies of our soul is revealed.
- His physical body gets the victory over the diseases of heart, brain, liver, lungs, spleen and kidney etc.

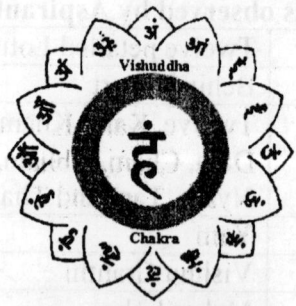

Vishuddha Chakra

Description of Vishuddha Chakra as observed by Aspirant

Shape	Sixteen petalled Lotus
Location	Behind Throat

Nadis	Sixteen: Am, Aam, Im, Eem, Um, Uum, Rshim, Reem, Lrim, Lreem, Eiym, Eeiym, Om, Aum, Am and Ah
Bija Mantra	Ham
Granthi	Vishnu Granthi
Loka	Janar Loka
Color of Nadis	Dark smoky
Vayu	Udana
Yantra	Round
Element/ color	Ether (Space) / Blue
Goddess	Shakini
God	Five Faced Lord Shiva
God Element	Cosmic
Animal	Elephant

What Happens When Vishuddha Chakra is opened?

- The opening of Vishuddha Chakra bestows the victory over the ether (space) element.
- The yogi is blessed with the Siddhi of reading the thoughts of others.
- A continuous tingling sensation at the back of the head is felt at *Bindu* Chakra.
- Yogi gets the knowledge of past, present and future.
- Brilliance radiance (Aura) is provided to the body.
- The yogi gets the victory over his hunger and can survive without any food and water for many days.
- The aspirant's soul is awakened from its eternal sleep and merges back into the cosmic energy.

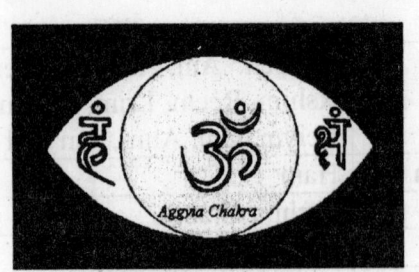

Aggyia Chakra

Description of Aggyia Chakra as observed by Aspirant

Shape	Two petalled Lotus
Location	Between the eye brows, behind forehead.
Nadis	Two. Ham, Ksham
Bija Mantra	Aum
Granthi	Rudra Granthi
Loka	Tapo Loka
Color of Nadis	White
Vayu	Apana, Vyana, Samana, Prana, Udana
Yantra	Round
Element/ color	Mind / Void
Goddess	Hakini
God	Shada-Shiva
God Element	Inverted Triangle
God Energy	Ishvara
Contrl. Deity	Rudra
Energy Centre	Inverted Triangle
Related Other Minor Chakras	Sixteen. Vishalaxmi, Vishnu-Maya, Vismalochana, Vriddhi, Yamabhagani, Yamaghanta, Yasa, Manotiga, Mati, Matrika, Mayavi, Mayuri, Madha, Maghvasini. Mohini and Muktakeshi

What Happens When Aggyia Chakra is opened

- The yogi remains in his undisturbed state of bliss & joy and the tingling sensation in chakras is stopped.
- His aura is transformed into an illuminating energy around the body.
- The aspirant gets an extraordinary radiance at his face.
- The yogi gets the power (siddhi of *Parkaya Pravesha*) of entering into the physical body of others.
- The yogi achieves victory over all the five elements: Earth, Water, Air, Fire, Ether and also his Consciousness & Mind.
- At this stage guidance of Guru is needed for lifting the Kundalini further to the Sahasrara.
- The aspirants experience Samadhi, which is the highest step in the eightfold step in *Yog-Sutras* of Maharishi Patanjali.

There are two types of main *Samadhies*. *Sabhikalpa Samadhi* (absorption with fluctuations) and *Nirvikalpa Samadhi* (absorption without any fluctuation). When the Kundalini pierces Aggyia chakra, *Sabhikalpa samadhi* is attained as the meditator, the process of meditation and the object of meditation become one with God. There are various stages of *Sabhikalpa samadhi*. The intermediate state between the two is called *Asampragyata samadhi* (absorption without awareness). It is difficult to differentiate the transition from *Sabhikalpa* to *Asampragyata* to *Nirvikalpa samadhi*, as it is difficult to differentiate when the youth ends and old age begins.

Swami Satyananda Saraswati in his book "Kundalini Tantra" page 204, has clarified the above situation as follows:

"The whole process occurs in continuity, each stage fusing into next and transforming in a very graduated way. This seems logical when you consider that it is the same consciousness which is undergoing the experience .....

From *Muladhara* upto Aggyia chakra, the awareness is experiencing higher things, but it is not free from ego. You cannot transcend ego at the lower points of awakening. It is only when Kundalini reaches Aggyia chakra that the transcendence begins. There is where the ego is exploded into a million fragments and the ensuing death experience occurs. At this point *Sabhikalpa* ends and *Nirvikalpa* begins. From here, the energies fuse and flow together up to *Sahasrara*, where enlightenment unfolds."

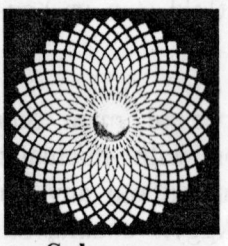

Sahasrara

Description of Sahasrara Chakra as observed by Aspirant

Shape	Thousand (*Sahasra*) petalled Lotus
Location	Top of the brain
Nadis	One Thousand Nadis one with each petal from 'A' to 'Ksa'
Bija Mantra	Param Shiva
Granthi	Beyond
Loka	Satya-Loka
Color of Nadis	Rainbow colors

Vayu	Beyond the realm of Vayus
Yantra	Full Moon
Color of the Element	In-Explicable
Goddess	Maha-Laxmi
God	Lord-Shiva
God Element	All the Gods & Goddesses are present in it.
God Energy	Jyotir Lingam
Contrl. Deity	Lord Shiva
Energy Centre	Moon
Related Other Minor Chakras	*Thousand minor chakras.* Nearly 25% minor chakras are related with physical body, 25% with etheric body and the rest with the spiritual progress of the aspirant.

There are seven more chakras beyond the realm of the *Sahasrara*. These are difficult to achieve by the ordinary aspirants. These chakras provide the ultimate knowledge of the entire manifested and the unmanifested Brahman (Lord Shiva in formless state). These are beyond the realm of the seven *Lokas* known to few. These chakras if opened provide the perfect realization of God. All these are above the *Sahasrara,* one over the other starting in the following sequence:

1. Narada Chakra
2. Ananta Chakra
3. Muktananda Chakra
4. Vyasa Chakra
5. Vyapini Chakra
6. Uthana Chakra
7. Uttarakashi Chakra

What Happens When Kundalini Crosses the Sahasrara

Sahasrara cannot be termed as a Chakra as it does not have a direct link with the physical body, but most of the people call it a Chakra. It is a reservoir of life-energy and Cosmic-energy. Like a UPS or inverter, it supplies immediate energy to the body in emergency need. It is difficult to describe the indescribable *Sahasrara*. The moment a yogi attains the realms of Sahasrara, he becomes beyond the comprehension of human knowledge. *It is rightly said, "He who knows, speaks not, and he who speaks, knows not."*

For a yogi it is the highest realm of spiritual achievement (*Nirvikalpa samadhi*). Sahasrara is also called as *Brahmarandhra* or *Kala* Chakra or *Shanta* Chakra.

The synonym Crown (***Lalta***) Chakra generally mentioned by the western writers is not exactly the Sahasrara. But it is little below the Sahasrara. The Crown Chakra is responsible for the etheric body of the yogi. On the other hand beyond the gross body is due to Crown chakra. The Crown (*Lalta*) Chakra does not have any particular shape. Its color changes with the change of color of other Chakras. It is just as the white light is refracted through a glass prism it is dispersed into seven or innumerable different colors. The Kundalini energy is also refracted into innumerable colors.

Sahasrara has one thousand petals and Nadis. It also reflects the various colors of other chakras. It confuses an aspirant to presume it as Lalta chakra. The Lalta chakra helps yogis to achieve the *Moksha or Nirvana* (freedom from birth & death). The advanced yogis are able to escape their soul through this chakra at the time of their death.

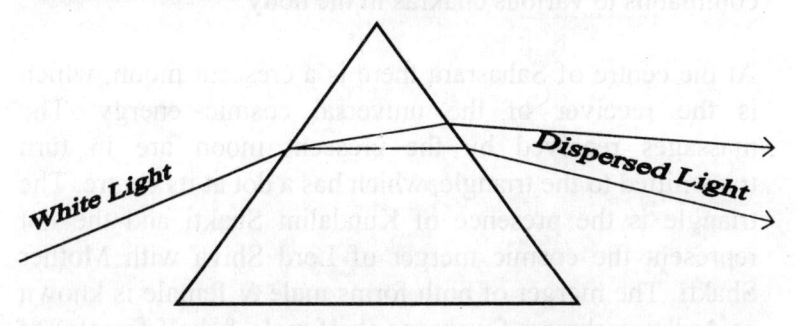

White Light is dispersed into Seven Colors by Glass Prism

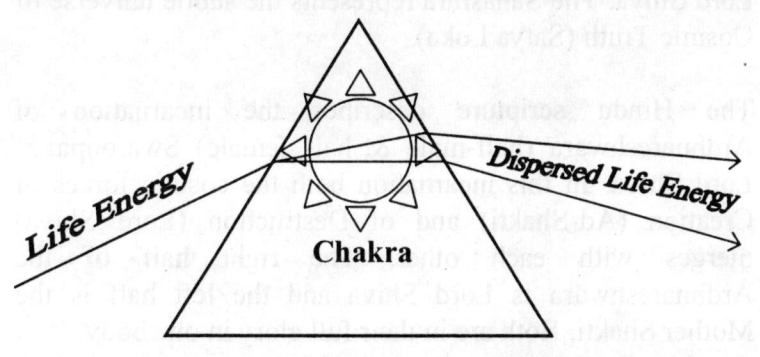

Cosmic Life Energy is dispersed into Many Sub-Pranic Energies by a Chakra inside the Spine

There are twenty different layers of petals one above the other in the Sahasrara. Each layer has fifty petals. In all there are thousand petals. Each layer of petals has a different color. A nadi is emanating out from each petal. These nadis are connected with other six main chakras in spine and with many minor chakras in the astral body.

Each nadi is associated with a particular sound of a different letter of Sanskrit. Each petal produces a different cosmic sound audible to the sensory preceptors and the nadis. These sounds are the signals of massages and commands to various chakras in the body.

At the centre of Sahasrara there is a crescent moon, which is the receiver of the universal cosmic energy. The massages received by the crescent moon are in turn transmitted to the triangle, which has a dot at its centre. The triangle is the presence of Kundalini Shakti and the dot represent the cosmic merger of Lord Shiva with Mother Shakti. The merger of both forms male & female is known as Ardhnareshwara Swaroopa (half male & half female) of Lord Shiva. The Sahasrara represents the subtle universe of Cosmic Truth (Satya Loka).

The Hindu scripture describes the incarnation of Ardhnareshwara (half-male & half female) Swaroopa of Lord Shiva. In this incarnation both the cosmic forces of Creation (Ad-Shakti) and of Destruction (Lord Shiva) merges with each other. The right half of the Ardhnareshwara is Lord Shiva and the left half is the Mother Shakti. Both are in their full glory in one body.

The moment Kundalini Shakti reaches Sahasrara; yogi loses his individuality and ego 'I'. His soul merges with the Cosmic Soul of God. His separate identity vanishes. He becomes one with God and gets all the powers like omnipotence, omniscient and omnipresence of God. This is known as self-realization or enlightenment. This is the ultimate goal of yoga and human life. God has given us the human body only to realize God.

At this stage the yogi merges his identity with Brahman and he can rightly say: 'Aham Brahmasmi', 'So-Ham' and 'Eko-Brahman Dityio Nahi'. In this absolute state of Brahman there are no laws of sciences governing matter, no relativity, no time, no place, no space, no creation, no matter, no energy, no day or night, no light or darkness, no present-past-future, no birth or death, no duality, no pain or pleasure and no happiness or sorrow. Only the Sat (Truth), Chit (Consciousness) and Ananda (Bliss) are left.

A yogi can hold and stay in this extraordinary state of consciousness for hours at a stretch. But the Kundalini Shakti may start its downward journey from Sahasrara to Muladhara, if the fruits of his past actions (samskaras) are not completely washed away. There is no doubt that a new kingdom is opened for the aspirant, but it is simply a visitor's visa for a short duration. It may take some time to become the citizen of the new country. The visitor visa may expire also.

That is why the Kundalini comes back to Muladhara because the fruits of the past actions (*Karamphals*) of the yogi are still not washed away. Unless all the fruits of past actions are completely washed away, the yogi cannot remains in the above absolute state forever. So along with the yog-sadhana (yoga-practice) a yogi must not ignore the Yama & Niyama as defined in the Holy Scriptures and these should not be diluted or twisted by any illogic as done by some of the modern authors (mostly westerners).

Nonetheless, there is a stage when every thing comes to an end and the tiny soul merges with ocean. At this stage all the interests of the realized yogi are lost and there remains no cause to continue to live in his present physical body. Such a realized saint predicts to leave his body to his disciples at a particular date and time. He takes his *Mahasamadhi* at the determined predicted time. There had been numerous instances of *Mahasamadhi* by the enlightened saints in India.

The Problems of Improper Awakening of Kundalini

Improper awakening of Kundalini is really a dangerous situation. It hampers the smooth life of the aspirant. Many bodily and mental problems may arise such as:
- Loss of confidence, anxiety and nervousness
- Lack of concentration, stress and mental depression
- Hostility and aggressiveness and suspicion to others
- Over-sex problems
- Conflict with the employer may arise which leads to psychosomatic illness

Does the Awakening of Kundalini means Self-Realization or Enlightenment

The awakening of Kundalini is not the end but the beginning of the spiritual journey for self-realization. Self-realization is the ultimate aim to achieve by all the yogis. But awakening is definitely a forward step toward the goal of self-realization. There cannot be any self-realization without the awakening and activation of the Kundalini. There are some exceptions that some may achieve self-realization without awakening of the Kundalini. But it is rare due to the mercy of God.

!Om Anandam Om!

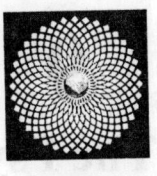

9

Granthis: The Psychic Knots

Prayer

Granthis: The Psychic Knots

Brahma Granthi

Vishnu Granthi

Rudra Granthi

9

Granthis: The Psychic Knots

Prayer

In the Ocean of Creation, O Ma Kali! I hear the rhythm of Thy footsteps of wild dance. Thousands of stars & galaxies are dancing and shining on Thy beauteous bosom. I am a tiny bubble of life in the vast Ocean of Creation (*Bhav-Sagar*), looking for Thy shore-less Shore. Help me to cross the Sea, O Mother Divine, to reach Thy Shore.

O Goddess Mother! Though art creating the infinite numerous dreams of creation, preservation and destruction. On the screen of Thy cosmic space, Thou art creating billions of cosmic dramas of your dreams in the minds of the tiny creatures.

O Mother of All! Make me free from the glittering veil of the enchanting dreams and the strong bond of the delusive *Maya*.

Granthis: The Psychic Knots

Granthis are the psychic knots of the nadis in the spinal chord; these are other than the chakras made up of the ethereal matter. Granthis play an important role in deciding the awakening of the Kundalini, *partially or fully*. Unless tackled tactfully, these become the biggest hurdle and hindrance in the upward journey of Kundalini. These Granthis (knots) are responsible to provide many *Siddhis* and *Riddhis* to aspirants, if opened and balanced properly. There are three major Granthis:

- *Brahma Granthi*
- *Vishnu Granthi*
- *Rudra (Mahesha) Granthi*

Brahma, Vishnu & Rudra (Mahesha) are the Trinity of God (*Adi-Purusha*) as per the Scriptures. These Knots (*Granthis*) are the main hindrance in the movement of the Kundalini energy upward. The Granthis are cosmic in nature and plays a vital role. The Granthis decide the full or the partial awakening in the opening of the six Chakras. The Granthis are also to be opened by the aspirant tactfully.

The knot of *Brahma* restricts the Muladhara chakra. The knot of *Vishnu* restricts the Anahata chakra and the knot of *Rudra* restricts the Aggyia chakra. These knots form an significant role in yogic practices and the stages toward enlightenment by breaking through these knots. As per the Scriptures, four stages of progress are described such as *arambha, ghata, parichaya* and *nishpatti*.

Arambha is associated with breaking the knot of *Brahma*. *Ghata* is associated with breaking the knot of *Vishnu*. *Parichaya* & *nishpatti* are associated with breaking the knot of *Rudra*. After balancing these knots Kundalini may ascend to Sahasrara.

Brahma Granthi

It is the first major blockage to surpass. Without opening of Brahma Granthis it is not possible to come out of the bondage of the material worldly things. This Granthi is linked to other four smaller Granthis. These are known as *Bhairavi, Vishala, Chamunda* and *Shirsha*. All these Granthis keep the men under the temptation and bondages of material things like money, lethargy, worldly pleasures, land, property, sex, and ignorance due to Maya. These characteristics develop the concept of Ego 'I' and selfishness in the human personality. After opening of this Granthis the temperature in the genital and anal region becomes little lesser then the body temperature. The Brahma-Granthi works as a thermostat for the lower parts of the body. The aspirant feels a tingling sensation in these areas. Brahma Granthi works as a Pre-Kundalini Awakening Syndrome.

The opening of Brahma Granthi may also cause many problems and troubles such as:
➢ Rise in body temperature
➢ Extreme sexual urge
➢ Extreme lust for material worldly things

But the benefits of opening of Brahma Granthi are much more and the aspirant should not be afraid of its opening:
➢ It also opens and channelises the three lower major chakras of the aspirant: Muladhara, Swadhisthan and Manipur.
➢ The aspirant is blessed with many siddhis and riddhis.

➢ The awakening of this Granthi restricts the activities of the: politicians, businessmen, moneylenders and the greedy-men.

Japa Exercise for Balancing the Brahma Granthi

Sit comfortably in your asana, better in the morning or evening. Place your right hand over the Anahat chakra and left hand over the Muladhara chakra. Inhale, retain and exhale your breath deeply in the ratio 1:2:3 and chant any one of the mantra

➢ Om Brahmayae Namah! or
➢ Om Anandam Om!

Mentally repeat these mantras as many times as you can. These mantras help in purifying this Granthi and allow the flow of cosmic energy smoothly. After the japa exercise, pray God for the balancing of this Granthi. Meditate for some time by concentrating your mind at this Granthis. A white shining cosmic energy is felt flowing from the top of the head (Medulla Oblongata) to the base of the body. While flowing down this energy splits into various strands of white color, just as a glass prism splits the white light or sunrays into many colors[1].

After the meditation, raise your hands in the *namaskar* mudra above your heart, prey God for the balancing of this Granthi.

Vishnu Granthi

Vishnu Granthi is the second major Granthi, which obstruct the aspirants from further progress. It belongs to Lord

---

[1] See the pictures of dispersion of light by prism and prana by chakras in this book.

Vishnu. This Granthi is related to four other important minor Granthis known as Shyamla, Krishna, Neelanjana, and Shanmukha. These smaller Granthis keep the aspirants under the wraps of attachments, inner psychic visions and emotional bondages. All these are the cause of selfishness and super-ego in human beings. Ego becomes so powerful that it keeps the aspirant attached to it and stops his further progress.

The opening of Vishnu Granthi bestows so many advantages like
- It energizes and channelises the Anahata & Vishuddha chakras.
- The aspirant is filled with divine love for all and becomes attractive to others. The aspirant gets the power to understand others without any verbal communication.
- Provides many types of siddhis and riddhis: like the creation of sacred ash and many things out of nothing.
- Te nadis in the region of Anahat chakra get cleansed and balances this Granthi.

The Vishnu Granthi restricts the further progress of the aspirants who are ruthless, inhuman and unsympathetic to others. So the aspirants must have to change themselves accordingly.

Even the opening of this Vishnu Granthi causes many problems & troubles. But once opened it remains open forever. The aspirant is filled with love for all. This love does not mean sexual love.

Many times the siddhis and riddhis leads to a false pride and obstructs achieving the ultimate goal. If so, the aspirant stops his practices and begins to lose his yogic achievements. Therefore one should ignore the riddhis and siddhis. But an *Avatara* (like Rama & Krishna) is an incarnation of God and does his *Lila* (actions not under the Karmic-Law). An Avatara has all riddhis and siddhis by birth and he is entitled to perform the miracles frequently to establish the faith of God in public, without any fear of loosing the spiritual powers. Avatara himself is God and not a human being.

Japa Exercise for Balancing the Vishnu Granthi

Sit comfortably on your asana, better in the morning or evening. Place your right hand over the Anahat chakra and the left hand over the Manipur chakra. After some time place your hands in Jnana Mudra. Inhale, retain and exhale your breath deeply in the ratio 1:2:3 and chant any one of the mantra
- Om Namo Naraayanayee Namah! or
- Om Namo Bhagwate Vasudevayae Namah!

Mentally repeat these mantras as many times as you can. After the japa exercise, pray God for the balancing of this Granthi. Meditate for some time by concentrating your mind at this Granthis it will be balanced.

Rudra Granthi

It is the third and last major Granthi to obstruct. It belongs to Lord Shiva. This Granthi obstructs the aspirants from further progress from crossing the tenth door. This Granthi is responsible for the hindrance for the opening of the Aggyia Chakra. Rudra Granthi is related to six important minor Granthis known as Roudra, Mukti, Sanathya, Kapali, Kalachudas and Kulashrva. All these smaller Granthis keeps the aspirant under the wraps of material attachments, illusions of riddhis and inner psychic powers.

This Granthi keeps the aspirant attached to it and stops his further progress. On balancing this Granthi the aspirant is blessed to attain the stage of *Nirvikalpa* samadhi and have the experience of the cosmic bliss of Shiva Shakti. This Granthi is very difficult to open by the aspirant himself. Only a self-Realized guru can help in opening this Granthi. A realized guru is needed at this stage for further progress.

The opening of Rudra Granthi bestows many powers, Riddhis and Siddhis like:
> The secret of creation of the universe is revealed to the aspirant. Aspirant is detached form the great illusion and delusion due to *Maya*. He comes closer to God-realization.
> Once opened this Granthi also remains opened for the lifetime.
> It provides many extraordinary *siddhis & riddhis*
> All the chakras are energized and channelised to connect with the Aggyia chakra.
> The emotions like anger, dullness, agony, sadness, happiness, fear and surprise are get away one after the other from the aspirant.
> Once opened, it also remains open for the lifetime.
> When this Granthi is opened, the aspirant gets a victory over the illusions, delusions and Maya of the world. He gets connected with the realm of God-Realization.

It is *tamsik* in nature. Many times the *riddhis* leads for the increase of a false pride of ego and increases desire for material things in the aspirant. Eight major siddhies and nine types of riddhis are gifted to the aspirant. If the aspirant stops his further practices, one day he may lose his yogic achievements. Therefore one should ignore these riddhis and siddhis, which are like the toys and toffees given to a child to distract his mind from the mother (real aim).

Japa Exercise for Balancing the Rudra Granthi

Sit comfortably on your asana, better in the morning or in the evening at sun-set. Place your left hand over the Anahat chakra and right hand over the Vishuddha chakra then after some time in Jnana Mudra. Inhale, retain and exhale your breath deeply in the ratio 1:2:3 and chant any one of the mantra

- Om Namo Rudraye Namah! or
- Om Anandam Om! or
- Om Namah Shivaya! or
- The following **Maha-Mritunjia Mantra**

Om Tri-yambakam Yajamahe Sugandhim Pushti Vardhanam! Urvaruk-mive Bandhanan Mritiyor Mokshyiam Amritat!!

Mentally repeat these mantras as many times as you can. After the japa exercise, pray God for the balancing of this Granthi and then meditate for some time by concentrating your mind at this Granthis. The opening of this Granthi increases the closeness of the aspirant with the Supreme Being. Aspirant is bestowed with comic bliss (Ananda).

! Om Anandam Om !

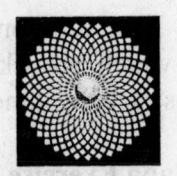

10
Shaktipat

Prayer

Initiation of Disciples by Shaktipat

Warning About *Shaktipat* by Quacks and Fakes

Restrictions for Shaktipat

10
Shaktipat

Prayer

O Universal Immortal Creative Power! Thou art Omniscient and All-pervading Ruler. Thou art alone the Protector from the powerful *Maya* in this illusive changeable universe. None else can exist in Thy imaginary dream universe, to govern this world eternally.

Thou art created the Holy Vedas and the Individual Kundalini Power, and gifted these to Thy loving children for seeking their liberation of soul from the clutches of the powerful *Maya*. Thou art the remover of all the sins, fruits of past karmas, attachments and ignorance. Enlighten our soul and intellect to merge in Thy Cosmic Sea. Awaken our dormant power of Kundalini hidden in our Muladhara to realize Thee.

Initiation of Disciples by Shaktipat

'*Shakti*' means 'energy' and '*pat*' means 'bestowing'. Shaktipat means '*bestowing the energy or lighting the lamps*'. Shaktipat is the transfer of energy for awakening of the Kundalini of the disciple by the grace of God and Guru. A realized Guru can awaken the Kundalini of the aspirant by the transfer of energy to the aspirant. *Shaktipat* activates the dormant Kundalini and is like the lighting a candle with another, which is already lit.

But there is a big question: Whether the aspirant should cleanse himself of the impurities and imperfections first and after that he is entitled for the initiation with Shaktipat or should the Shaktipat be done first and then after the body, nadis, intellect and mind are cleansed?

The initiation along with Shaktipat is a rare blessing of a Guru. There are only very few realized Gurus entitled for this debatable issue: as to whether the initiation with Shaktipat is possible? Even if fortunately you meet such a Guru by the grace of God, there are chances that you would not be able to recognize him, unless the true Guru desires so. Even if you recognize him and also willing to accept him as your Guru, there is no guarantee that the realized Guru will accept you as his disciple. Also the initiation with *Shaktipat* is not for everyone. A true Guru is also not entitled to initiate all his disciples by the process of *Shaktipat*. If a Guru claims so, he may be a fake Guru.

The scriptures have laid down many essential qualifications for an aspirant to become worthy of the grace of the Guru for Shaktipat. The *Mundaka Upanishad* warns us "*Unless a disciple has achieved the difficult task such as of carrying fire upon his head, his Spiritual Teacher (Guru) should not impart the mystic knowledge to him."* Again the *Upanishads* (Holy Scriptures) also advise us *"The mystic knowledge may be imparted to a worthy disciple, who has already lived with his Guru for quite a long time, and has done his best efforts to achieve God-realization."*

A disciple himself is not competent to estimate the worthiness of his deserving for the Shaktipat by his Guru. It is the true Guru, who really knows through his inner spiritual 'third eye' and the intuitive power, about the spiritual progress and eligibility of his disciple for the Shaktipat. The disciple should be in benevolent protection of a perfect master (true Guru), who can easily watch and keep a control over the movement of the Kundalini through the chakras of his disciple. The disciple should be under his direct check to avoid any mishap. Otherwise it can be a horrifying and painful experience, unless one has purified and perfected his body, mind and nadis through the scientific yoga practices.

During the Mahabharata, Lord Krishna imparted the mystic divine knowledge of yoga (Bhagwad Geeta) to his disciple Arjuna. But the Arjuna found him undeserving for this. He reportedly said to Krishna, *"None of the sign or symptom of a saint or a yogi is in me. I feel myself unworthy of the essentials of yogic requirements for such a divine knowledge, yet I shall try my best to be able to achieve this through your grace."*

Lord Krishna put a counter question to Arjuna and asked, *"Can anybody obtain the divine knowledge of the Almighty God without deserving on the part of the doer?"* This question itself affirms that the Lord had already judged the inherent ability of his disciple Arjuna, with His Supreme intuitive power. Without achieving the requirement of deserving ability one cannot know and contact with God.

It is strange that the *Sufis* and many other sects believe that the Shaktipat can be done first, without fulfilling the condition of deserving ability of the disciple. According to them it can be given to any body at any time, whether someone is interested in God or not. Their argument to justify is: "It is not possible by man to purify his mind and nadis, without first illuminating his Spirit. The own efforts of a disciple by his yogic practices cannot cleanse his body, mind and nadis. But the transfer of energy by a Guru to his disciple, through the grace of God can cleanse the disciple".

This logic seems to be false and distorted. I strongly disagree with this opinion. If it is true, then a Guru can initiate by Shaktipat any number of men in the world, even without asking for their initiation and then by this way the Kundalini of all the men in the world can be awakened easily by a Guru, which will cleanse every body automatically. It is against the will of God due to His Maya. Since it has never happened in the past and it will never happen in future also.

A real Guru can't go against the will of God. Shaktipat on a mass-scale claimed by so many so-called modern Gurus is a fake activity and it is not possible by them. Shaktipat is only possible with a disciple, who has gone through a long period of his great efforts, discipline, austerity, and spiritual practices. A disciple may be ready for initiation only when he has done his *Sadhana* with all the sincerity, faithfulness and truthfulness. At the right time God sends a true master (Guru) for his proper initiation to remove the spiritual obstacle in the disciple.

The awakening of the Kundalini is a most auspicious event like the birth and the death, in the life of a man. But it will be of no use if the aspirant does not practice long meditation and follow all the Yama & Niyama as given in the scriptures and not distorted or twisted by any one.

Kundalini can be awakened in many ways, such as attaining perfection in *asanas*, *pranayama*, meditation and intense devotion. Also by the grace of God and by Shaktipat a realized Guru can transmit life-energy to an aspirant and awaken his Kundalini. This can be accomplished in four ways: by touch; gaze; mantra and thought transfer. The Guru may touch the disciple and transmit energy through physical contact, or gaze at the disciple so that energy flows from the Guru's eyes. The Guru may utter powerful mantra, which transfers life-energy to the disciple, or the life-energy can be transferred directly by the Guru through his thought or will.

Once the Kundalini is awakened, the disciple may have a variety of experiences: He may see flashes of light or colors, hearing internal sounds of bells ringing or bees humming, spontaneous vibrations in body, or movements in the body, or greater mental peace, to name a few. Different individuals will have different experiences after awakening of Kundalini. There is no definite pattern applicable to everyone. Once the Kundalini is awakened, the aspirant goes through his own experiences to realize this fact. If at this stage the aspirant practices deep meditation, then the Kundalini will travel upward from the Muladhara to Aggyia chakra.

It has been noted that the piercing of chakras by the Kundalini may not be in a sequence from the Muladhara to Aggyia chakra. Any of the chakra can become active first and any of the chakra can become activated in the last. When a chakra is activated a lot of life-energy gets stored therein and the aspirant experiences an extreme hotness in the region. By the accumulation of energy at the chakra, a sort of brilliant 'sun' shines inside the chakra. But when the Kundalini leaves the chakra it becomes just lifeless and an extreme coldness is felt.

Since the accumulated fruits of the past actions (karmas) are different for everybody, therefore the yoga practice of any two persons in the world is also different and can never be the same. Similarly the awakening of the Kundalini experience of no two persons can ever be the same.

Warning About *Shaktipat* by Quacks and Fakes

A *Shaktipat* is not an exclusive and separate branch of yoga. Many ignorant and layman neo-spiritual teachers and authors are twisting the ancient Hindu Scriptures and claiming it as something special and different from other yoga systems. We know that energy always flows from higher potential to lower potential. The *Shaktipat* is the technique of awakening the Kundalini of an *eligible, mature and deserving disciple* by a self-realized Guru, by transferring his life force at a higher potential level to a deserving disciple whose life force is at a lower potential level. This is purely with the grace of an authorized Guru in very special circumstances. Even the Guru like Rama-Krishna Paramhansa did not frequently used this technique on his disciples; otherwise he would have awakened the Kundalini of millions of people in the world. God do not permit his saints to violate His spiritual laws.

Shaktipat

Never think that the great spiritual Gurus of ancient India were not aware of the awakening of the Kundalini by *Shaktipat*, as some of the ignorant, fake & self-declared gurus claim these days that they can awaken the Kundalini of any number of person even from a remote distance, without any eligibility criteria of the disciple and further his disciples can also do the same to others. In fact even the Kundalini of such Gurus is not awakened. How can they awaken the Kundalini of others? They do not know, what Kundalini awakening is? If their claim is true then the ancient Gurus who were much more spiritually advanced must have awakened the Kundalini of all the people in the world, without any difficulty.

Simply awakening of the Kundalini does not mean it is active also and it is not the ultimate aim of yoga. The ultimate aim of Kundalini awakening is self-realization. Never accept any body as your spiritual Guru unless you are sure he is self-realized and not a fake Guru.

Restrictions for Shaktipat

As per the Holy Scriptures, the following restrictions, which must be observed both by the aspirant and his Gurus:
- Guru must be self-realized i.e. whose Kundalini is already awakened, active and has pierced all the chakras including Sahasrara.
- The disciple must be eligible and a deserving candidate for Shaktipat i.e. he has already purified his body, mind, nadis and intellect as defined by the scriptures.
- It is better if the disciple live personally with his Guru in his ashram some time before and after the awakening of the Kundalini.

- ➢ The disciple has been regular in his yoga practices for quite a long time but he himself is not able to awaken his Kundalini, due to some unknown reasons.
- ➢ The Guru should know the real cause of the hindrance of not awakening of the Kundalini of his disciple by his intuitive knowledge (Third Eye).
- ➢ The awakening of the Kundalini is not possible from a distance or by post or by any communication or in a mass-scale as a group activity. If a Guru claims so, it is certainly misleading.
- ➢ After the Shaktipat the Guru should have the spiritual power to control the problems, which may arise by the forceful awakening of the Kundalini of the disciple.

!Om Anandam Om!

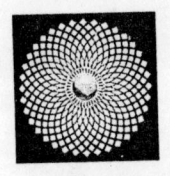

11

Important Powerful Mantras & Yantras

Prayer for Kundalini Shakti

Mantras for Awakening the Kundalini

The Chanting of Mantras for Worshiping of:
Brahman, Vishnu, Shiva, Guru
Ma Devi Durga and Ganesha

Mantras for Pacifying the Effect of Nine Planets (Graha)

Single Mantra for the Worship of The Nine Planets

Separate Mantras for Nine Planets:
Mantras for Sun (Surya), Moon (Chandra), Mars (Mangal), Mercury (Buddha), Jupiter (Guru), Venus (Shukra), Saturn (Shani), Rahu and Ketu

Mantra for Peace

Mantra for Joy & Bliss

Maha Gayatri Mantra

Other Mantras

11
Important Powerful Mantras & Yantras

Prayer for Kundalini

Om Jagatjanani Maa!
Om Mooladhara Vasini Maa!!
Uthana Uthana Uthana !!!
Om Kundalini Shaktiye Namah!

Mantras for Awakening the Kundalini

Mantras are the special words from the scriptures in Sanskrit, which have a great mystic spiritual power, when repeated mentally or orally during the concentration and meditation. Mantras should not to be translated in other languages, but it is better to understand their meaning before the japa. The repetition of mantra for some time is called Japa. Mantras have the power of the divine in the form of sound, word and letters. Mantras are the true instruments for getting rid of worldly fetters.

Awakening of Kundalini is affected by Mantra also. Japa is a part of Bhakti Yoga. The aspirants should repeat the Mantra if given by their Guru hundreds of time. During the time of Diksha of an aspirant, the Guru generally utters a sacred Mantra to his disciple. The Kundalini of some may awaken immediately. A Guru can raise the consciousness of the disciple to a high degree. This depends upon the faith of disciple in Guru and in the power of Mantra. Mantras, when received from the Guru in person have very powerful effect.

The aspirants in Kundalini and Kriya Yoga should take the *Mantra-Sadhana* only after getting a proper Mantra from a Guru. Therefore I am not touching this point in detail. Mantras when learnt through ordinary friends or through books do not produce much benefit. Mantras are numerous and by intuition Guru should select a specific Mantra, which is more useful to a particular disciple to awaken his Kundalini.

The Chanting of Mantras:

As per the scriptures, the first manifestation of Brahman in the human form is the Trinity (*Brahma, Vishnu and Mahesh*). They are known as *Adi-Purusha*.

For Worshiping Brahman:
Om is known as *Pranava* Mantra.
Om Brahmayae Namah!!
Sat-Chit-Anand Brahma Swaroopaaye Namah!!

Om Poornam-Madaa,Poornam-Midam,Poornat-Poorna-Mudachiate!
Poornasia, Poorna-Madaya,Poorna-Meva-Visisyiate!!
... *Isho-Upnishada*

This means: O, God! Thou art infinite and complete. Out of Thy infinite formless existence, the infinite creation (universe) has come out from Thee as Thou manifestation. Thou art (the left-after) is still infinite i.e. nothing has been reduced from Thee. Nothing can be added to Thee.

Important Powerful Mantras & Yantras

For Worshiping Vishnu:-

Om Namo Bhagvate Vasu-Devayai!!
Om Namo Narayanaye!!
Om!
Shanta-akaram, Bhujang-shaynam, Padam-nabham, Suresham!
Vishv-adharam, Gagan-sadrisham, Megh-Varnam, Shubhangam!.
Lakshmi-Kantam, Kamal-Nayanam, Yogirbhe-Dhyain-Gamiam!
Vande Vishnu, Bhav-Bhaya-Haranam, Sarve-Lokiak-Natham!!

Meaning:-

Shanta: Peaceful	Akaram : Form	Bhujang: Snake
Shayanam: Sleeping	Padam : Lotus	Nabham: Naval
Suresham: Lord of the gods.	Vishve: World	Adharam: Base
Gagan: Sky	Sadrisham: Equivalent	Megh: Cloud
Varnam: Form & color	Shubhngam: Auspisious	Laxmi: Goddess of wealth
Kantam: Glorified	Kamal: Lotus	Nayanam: Eyes
Yogir: Yogis	Dhyan: Meditation	Gamiam: Come in
Vande: Worship	Bhav: World	Bhaya: Fear
Haranam: who removes	Sarave: All	Lokiak Austral worlds
Natham: Lord		

For Worshiping Shiva:

Om Namah Shivaya!!

Om Sada-Shivaye Namah!!

Om Shivoham! Shivoham!! Shivoham!!!

Om Namo Rudraaye Namah!!

Maha Mrituanjia Mantra is most important mantra for curing the diseases and to release the soul from the physical body, without any pain at the time of death.

Om Tri-yambakam Yajamahe Sugandhim Pushti Vardhanam!
Urvarukmive Bandhanan Mritiyor Mokshyiam Amritat!!

Meaning: "I bow to the three-eyed Lord Shiva, who is always full of sweet fragrance, who nourishes the human beings. May He liberate me from the bondage of the enchanting world and death, just as a ripen fruit is naturally separated (without any pain) from the tree."

For Worshiping Guru:

Gurur Brahma, Gurur Vishnu; Guru Devo Mahashwara!
Gurur Sakchahat Parambrahamaha;
Tasmaii Sri Gurve Namaha!!

Om!
Brahamandam, Param Sukhdam; Kevalam Gyan Moortim!
Dwanda-teetam, Gagan Sadrisham; Tatvam-asi-adi Lakshanam!!
Ekam, Nityam, Vimalam, Achalam; Sarv-adhi-Sakashi Bhutam!
Bhavateetam, Tri-guna Rahitam; Sad-gurum Tam Namami!!

Meaning:
Brahamandam: Permanent Ananda (Bliss) of Brahman (God), Param: (Supreme), Sukhdam: giver of the pleasures, Kevalam: only, Gyan: knowledge, Moortim: an idol of worship. Dwanda-teetam: away form all kinds of dualities, Gagan: sky/space, Sadrisham: equivalent, Tatvamasi: God like, Adi-Lakshanam: qualities of God. Ekam: only one, Nityam: who is permanent & eternal, Vimalam: totally pure, Achalam: immovable, Sarvadhi: present everywhere, saakshi; witness, Bhutam: atma or soul, Bhawateetam: away from all kinds of emotions, Tri:

three, Guna: qualities or properties, Rahitam: devoid off, Sadgurum: self-realized guru, Tam: you, Namami: I bow my head at thy feet.

For Worshiping Divine Mother (Ma Devi Durga):

Om Sarve Mangal Maangalyie, Shive Sarvarth Sadhike! Sharaniye Triambake Gori Narayani Namostute!!

Om Shaktiaye Namah!

For Worshiping Goddess Maha Laxmi:

➢ *Om Maha Laxmiye Namah!*

For Worshiping Lord Ganesha

➢ *Om Ganapataye Namah!!*

➢ *Vakratunda Mahakaya Koti-Surya Samaprabhu! Nirvighnam Kurume Deva Sarva Karyeshu Sarvada!!*

➢ *Om Hum Glom, Haridrayae Ganpate, Var-Varad, Sarve-Janam, Hirdiyam Stambham Satmbham Swaha!!*

Mantras for Pacifying the Effect of Nine Planets (Graha)

The nine astrological planets have a great effect on our life activities and the fruits of karmas. The influence of the planet may be in our favor or against us. It is advisable for a wise man to control and increase the influence of the planets in his favor and to restrict and reduce the influence against him. The astrologers advise so many ways to control the influence. But the most important and the best is the repetition of particular mantra (japa) for the planet. Astrologically the Sun is also considered as a planet.

Single Mantra for the Worship of all The Nine Planets

Brahma Murari-s-Tripurant-Kari, Bhanu,
Shashi, Bhoomi Suto Budhascha!
Gurus-cha Shukra Shani Rahu Ketvah
Kurvantu Sarvemam Su-Prabhaatam!!

Separate Mantras for the Worship of The Nine Planets

1. Mantra for Sun (*Surya*)
Om Uditae Namah!

Om Uditaai Namah!

Om Udvidayai Namah!!

Om Japa Kusum, Sankashum Kashipeya Maha Dyutim!
Tamo-ari Sarv Paapghanam Pranato-asmi Divakaram!!

1. Mantra for Moon (*Chandra*)
Dadhi Shanka Tushaa-Rabham, Khseero Darnava Sambhavam!
Namaami Shashinam Somam, Shambhor Mukut Bhushanam!!

2. Mantra for Mars (Mangal)
Dharnee Garbha Sambhootam, Vidyut Kanti Samprabham!
Kumaram Shakti Hastam, Tam Mangalam Pranamamyam!!

3. Mantra for Mercury (Buddha)
Priyangu Kalika Shyaamam, Rupenda Pratimam Budham!
Soumyam Soumya Guno Pitam, Tam Budham Pranamamyam!!

5. Mantra for Jupiter (Guru)

Devanam Cha Rishi Naam Cha, Gurum Kanchan Sambhavam!
Buddhi Bhutam Trilokisham, Tam Namami Brihaspatim!!

6. Mantra for Venus (Shukra)
Him Kundaa Mrinaalabham, Daityanaam Patamam Gurum!
Sarv Shastra Pravaktaaram, Bhurgavem Paranaamyam!!

7. Mantra for Saturn (Shani)
Neelanjan Samaabhasam Ravi, Putram Yama Agrajam!
Chaaya Martand Sambhootam, Tam Namaami Shanaicharam!!

8. Mantra for Rahu
Ardha Kayam Maha Veeryam, Chandraditya Vimardanam!
Singhika Janani Sambhootam, Tam Rahu Pranamaayam!!

9. Mantra for Ketu
Palaash Pushpa Sankaasham, Taraka Graha Mastakam!
Rudram Rudraatmakam Ghoram, Tam Ketum Pranamaamyam!!

Mantras for Peace
Om Shanti! Shanti! Shanti!!

Om Peace! Peace! Peace!!

Mantras for Bliss & Joy
Om Anandam Om!
Om Anandam Om!!
Om Anandam Om!!!

Maha Gayatri Mantra
➢ *Om, Bhur Bhuva Swaha Tat Savitur Vaarenium!*
Bhargo Devsiya Dhimahi Dhiyo Yo Na Parchodyat!!

Meaning:
Om: Name of the Lord, Bhur: Physical World, Bhave: Astral World, Swaha: Celestial World, Tat: who

transcendents God, Savitura: who is a Creator, Vaarenium: who is adorable, Bhargo: who burns our sins or remove ignorance, Devasiya: Who is like God, Dheemahi: on whom I meditate, Dhio: with my intellect, Yo: which, Nah: us, Prachodyat: Enlighten us through your guidance.

Other Mantras

Om Asto Ma Sad-Gamiya!
Tamso Ma Jyotir-Gamaya!!
Mirtyior Ma Amritan-Gamyia!!!

Meaning: O Lord! Lead me from the path of untruth to truth, take me from darkness (ignorance) to light (knowledge) and take me from death (mortality) to the nectar of life (immortality).

Chanting-mantras to be repeated many times:

- *So-Ham! So-Ham! So-Ham!* ....
- *Om Guru! Om Guru! Om Guru!* ....
- *Om Krishan! Om Krishan! Om Krishan!* ....
- *Om Shivoham! Shivoham! Shivoham!* ....

SRI YANTRA

Meditation on Sri Yantra
The Wheel of Fortune

Yantras are the magical diagrams or geometrical figures used in Tantra worship. These are made from linear elements intended to represent in a synthetic form, the basic energies of the Nature, which are deities. They are the visual equivalents of the mantras or thought forms. A Yantra has a Mantra as its soul. Yantra is a three-dimensional figure and should be conceived as solid.

The most famous Yantra is Sri Yantra, which is known as "Wheel of Fortune". One should fix the picture of Sri Yantra on the wall in front of the meditation sitting posture. Concentrate and meditate on the Yantra for some time daily. It is useful to achieve good fortune.

Fix a large picture of this Yantra on the wall and Meditate

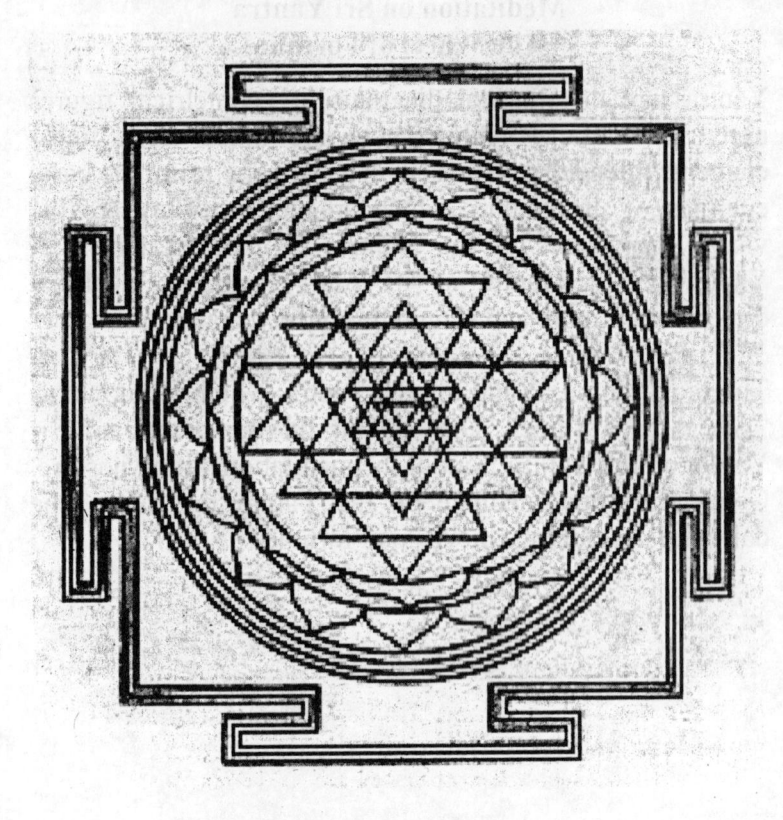

SRI YANTRA

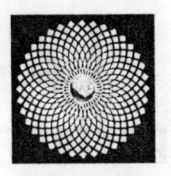

12
Useful & Important Information

How to become the member of the SRFY

Evolution of Five Gross Elements from Brahman

Dissolution of Five Gross Elements into Brahman

Five Basic Pranas

The Nine Main Elements in the Living Beings

Vital Energies their Regions & Responsible for

The Gross Body's Main Elements

The Gross Elements Produces Further Characteristics

Self-Realization Foundation of Yoga (SRFY)
Aims & Ideals
How to become the member of GRF

12
Useful & Important Information

Evolution of Five Gross Elements from Brahman

¶The Creation and Dissolution are the most important function of the Brahman. Everything has come out of Brahman. In the Scriptures the five gross elements Earth, Water, Fire, Air and Space (Ether) has not the same meaning as these are understood in sciences. These have much wider meanings as explained earlier.

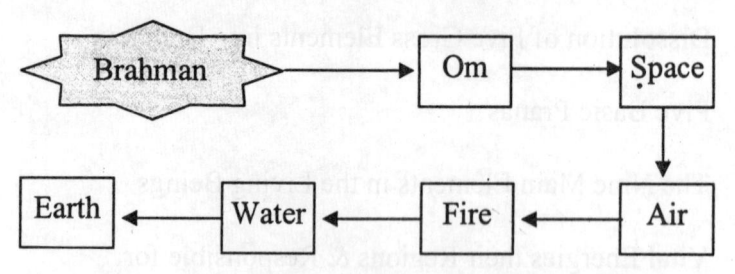

Brahman → Om → Space → Air → Fire → Water → Earth

Evolution of Five Gross Elements From Brahman

Dissolution of Five Gross Elements from Brahman

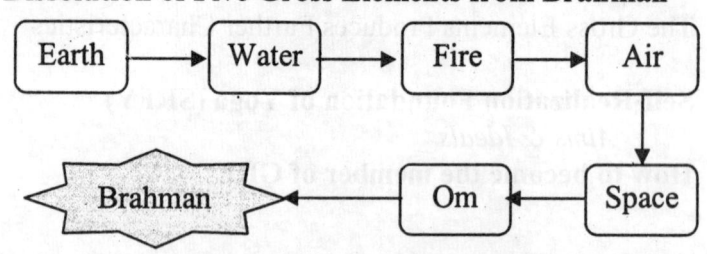

Earth → Water → Fire → Air → Space → Om → Brahman

Dissolution of Five Gross Elements into Brahman

---

[1] For details read the book "God and Self-Realization (Scientific and Spiritual View) by the same Author.

Five Basic Pranas
(Prana, Udana, Vyana, Samana, and Apana)
Each Prana has further five sub-pranas.

The Nine Constituents of Living Beings

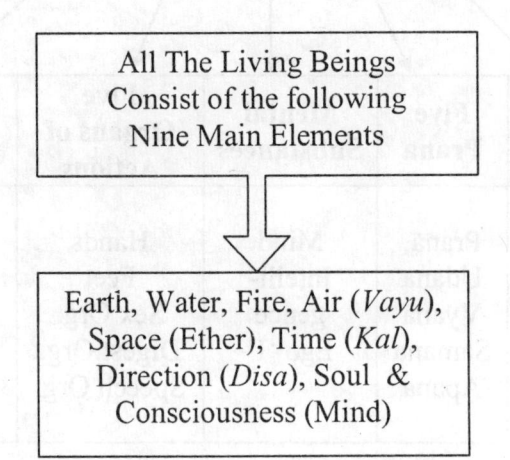

> All The Living Beings Consist of the following Nine Main Elements
>
> ⬇
>
> Earth, Water, Fire, Air (*Vayu*), Space (Ether), Time (*Kal*), Direction (*Disa*), Soul & Consciousness (Mind)

Vital Energies their Regions & Responsible for

Nine Main Vital Energies	The Region & Responsible for Play
Prana	Anus
Samana	Navel
Udana	Throat
Vyana	Throughout the body
Naga	It moves Upward
Kurma	Tirthas
Krikara	For Crying
Devadatta	For Yawning
Dhananjaya	For Singing & Roaring

```
                    ┌───────────┐
                    │ Gross Body │
                    └───────────┘
```

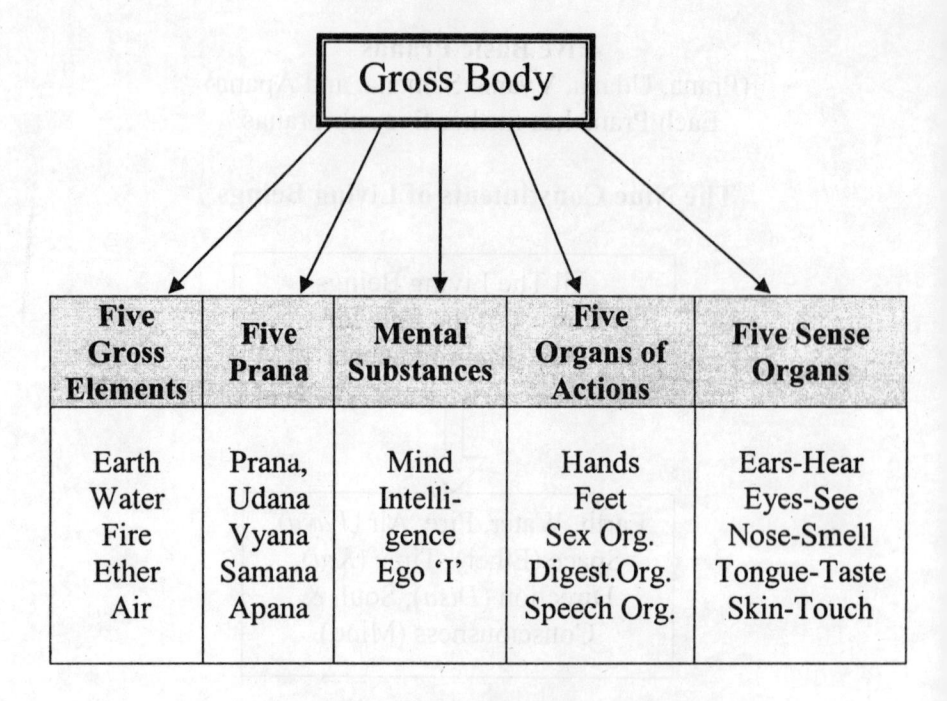

Five Gross Elements	Five Prana	Mental Substances	Five Organs of Actions	Five Sense Organs
Earth	Prana,	Mind	Hands	Ears-Hear
Water	Udana	Intelli-	Feet	Eyes-See
Fire	Vyana	gence	Sex Org.	Nose-Smell
Ether	Samana	Ego 'I'	Digest.Org.	Tongue-Taste
Air	Apana		Speech Org.	Skin-Touch

Further Characteristics Produced by Gross Elements

Elements	Characteristics
Space	Temptation, Desire, Anger, Delusion, Shame, Greed and Depression etc
Air	Knowledge, Concentrating, Expanding, Shaking, Throwing and Holding etc.
Fire	Thirst, Hunger, Fatigue, Sleep, Idleness, Pain and Tension etc.
Water	Blood, Urine, Faeces, Semen, Marrow, Phlegm & all the Fluids etc.

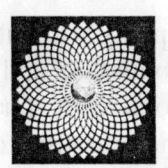

God-Realization Foundation (GRF) Aims & Ideals

It is a time for spiritual explosion of knowledge. Man has started thinking and seeking to know God for peace, joy and harmony. But man has also become extremely busy with his responsibilities of life. The explosion in Internet and communication Technology has solved this limitation of time. As such an organization like 'The God-Realization Foundation' (GRF) is very much needed in the busy world. The seekers of God need not wait for a Spiritual Guru, which is difficult to find also. You can get the required guidance and spiritual knowledge just at the click of button of your computer. To achieve this aim, GRF has been established by M/s. Geeta International Publishers & Distributors in India. Sh. Dharam Vir Mangla along with other spiritually advanced members has founded GRF to achieve its aims.

Its aims and ideals of GRF are:

➢ To provide e-spiritual technical guidance directly at home to the seekers of God, who are unable to join an Ashram personally in the company a Guru, leaving his family, office or business to suffer.
➢ To create love and devotion for God in the world.
➢ To provide the true universal broad concept of God and to remove the misconceptions about God by the sciences. To encourage the scientists to speak their

opinion and truth openly without fear to the world, who are till now silent about God and the Scriptures.
- To suggest new topics for further researches in the spiritual field for the scientists, doctors and technicians on the mystic scriptures and about miraculous powers and siddhis shown by the saints.
- As yoga is a universal science for all, the teachings of GRF are secular, universal, non-political and unbiased to any religion or philosophy.
- To answer the spiritual questions of its members and circulate it to other members, if it is useful to all.
- To conduct e-Spiritual-Achievements Tests for its members after every six months, so that they are able to know their achievements. After qualifying two tests, a member is entitled to receive Kriya-Yoga Initiation (Diksha). Then he will receive detailed knowledge of Kriya technique as given by Maharishi Patanjali. Before this eligibility Kriya practice will not be of much benefit.
- To provide more information about the miraculous saints and Holy Scriptures to its members.
- To serve the mankind and to bring a spiritual revolution in the world to bring peace, harmony, joy and ananda in the world.

How to become the member of GRF

Membership fee is Indian Rs. 450/- or US $ 10.0 per year. For registration, please send a crossed cheque or a demand draft in favor of 'Geeta International Publishers and Distributors' and inform your e-mail I-D, through e-mail dvmangla@hotmail.com. You will be allotted registered a membership number for all the facilities available under it.

Glossary

Advaita or Advaita	The viewpoint that consciousness can transcend duality and man can merge with God. There is only Brahman & nothing else. God & I are one & the same thing.
Aggyia Chakra	The Chakra between eyebrows.
Ahankar	Ego or 'I' associated with physical body. Also the false pride of ego.
Aham-Brahmashmi	I am God, or God and 'I' are one.
Ahankar	Egoism
Ahimsa	Non-injury, avoidance of violence, harmless.
Akasha or ether	Ether or space, first of five elements evolved from *Brahman (Om)*, the subtlest form of matter.
Amrita	Nectar of the gods, which makes the body immortal, an ambrosial liquid sometimes materialized by Sai Baba.
Anahat Chakra	The Chakra behind the throat (Cardiac plexus). One listens Anahat sounds on its opening.
Anahat Sounds	The inner sounds without any viberation of physical thing, audible even if you close your ears.
Ananda	Bliss, joy. Bliss is considered to be the very substance of God (God is bliss, not has bliss).
Ananda-Swaroopa	The very form of nature of bliss and *Ananda*.
Andhakoop	Dark well.
Arjuna	The disciple of Lord *Krishna* to whom *Krishna* revealed the truth of human existence just prior to the opening battle of the *Mahabharata* war. The divine is course is known as the *Bhagavad-Gita*.

Asana	Easy comfortable sitting posture. *Hatha yoga* posture of human body.
Ashanti	Grief, anxiety (absence of peace).
Ashram	Hermitage or monastery.
Astral body	Man's subtle body of light or prana or life force; Man has got three bodies: causal body, astral body and physical body. The astral body has nineteen elements: intelligence ego, feeling, mind, five senses, five instruments of actions, and five instruments of life force.
Astral-world	The subtle sphere of lord's creation, A universe of light and color composed of life energy or lifetrons. The subtlest aspect of one's being. That which is without any changes, unmodified, unaffected and timeless.
Atma	Individual soul; atma is the unseen basis, the substance of the entire objective world. It is the reality behind the appearance, universal and immanent in every being.
Atam-Shakti	The force and the power of the soul.
Atom	Basic unit of elements of ordinary matter
Avatar or Avatara	An incarnation of God. When God takes human form and play lila.
Avataran	The embodied lifetime of the *Avatar*. Descent of God in human form.
Avidya or Maya	Ignorance. Non-Knowledge.
Aum (Om)	The Cosmic sound Aum, which creates and sustains every thing. It is the Word or Holy Ghost or Hum or Amin.
Baba	Grand Father. A holy saint or *Sanyiasi*.
Belief	A hypothesis assumed to be true without verifying its truth.

GLOSSARY

Bhagavad-Gita or Geeta — This means "Song of the Lord". This is the renowned ancient scripture of India & part of the great epic *Mahabharata*. It has eighteen chapters and 700 *slokas*. It contains the spiritual teachings in the form of a dialogue between Lord *Krishna* to *Arjuna* (his disciple) *nearly 3250* years B.C., and is meant for all mankind. A must for all Yogis.

Bhagavan — Lord. God. "He who possesses all opulences".

Bhajan — Devotional songs.

Bhakta / Bhakti — A *bhakta* is a devotee, one who has *bhakti* (devotion), virtue, self-control, faith, and devotion to God.

Big-bang — The big explosion at the beginning of the universe in the singularity at the beginning of the universe in which the matter of the whole universe was condensed at a point of infinite density and gravitation. It was the beginning of the time.

Big-Crunch — The singularity at the end of the universe, when the matter of the whole universe is began to concentrate at infinite density and gravitation at a point.

Black hole — A region of space-time from which nothing can escape out, even the light and other waves cannot escape due to the huge force of gravitation.

Brahma — The creator God of the Hindu Trinity, the other two being Vishnu and Shiva.

Brahman	The ultimate, unchanging, Absolute Spirit composed of pure being and consciousness before the creation. The immanent principle, said to have three aspects: creation, preservation, and destruction. The absolute supreme reality Brahman is behind the apparent multiplicity of the phenomenal world.
Brahmachari	One who is a celibate
Brahmacharya	Celibacy
Buddhi	The discriminating faculty of mind, intellect, or intelligence.
Causal body	The man as a soul is a causal bodied being. The causal body is composed of 35 idea elements: 19 elements of the astral body + 16 basic elements of the physical body
Chakra	Seven spiritual centers or 'lotuses' of potential energy arrayed upward in man's ethereal or astral body from the base of the spine to the crown of the head.
Chit	Knowledge
Chitta	Subconscious mind
Darshan	See a great person and receive his blessing.
Death	When soul leaves the body permanently & four pranas also leave the body.
Delusion	Dual-vision, An illusion suffered by the whole humanity
Desires	Wish for, longing
Devotion	Love for seeking God.
Dharma	Religion of God, Righteousness, duty, code of conduct one of the four ends of human pursuit.
Dharana	Determination

GLOSSARY

Dhristrashtra	Father of Kaurvas in Mahabharata.
Dhyana	Meditation. The state of thoughtless consciousness with awareness of ego 'I'.
Diksha	Spiritual initiation, to dedicate oneself.
Dream	When mind completely detach itself from physical body and the ego creates another body & universe for itself.
Dus-karmas	Misdeeds, Bad-karmas.
Dwapara Yuga	See Treta Yugas.
Electron	A very small particle, which have negative charge that orbits the nucleus of the atom with a great velocity.
Elementary or subatomic particles	The particles which are believed to be further undivided like electron, proton, neutron, photon and many others.
Ether	It does not mean the ordinary organic chemical. The space between the heavenly bodies and the sub-atomic particles is not vacuum but it is filled with something throughout the universe and even inside the matter and particles. The whole universe is suspended in ether. Electromagnetic waves or light waves cannot travel in vacuum needs a medium, which is ether. It is the first and finest manifestation of God in the form of matter and all the subatomic particles has come out of it. It is still undetectable by the scientists.

Faith	An unshakable hypothesis presumed to be true, even it is failed.
Field	Something that exists throughout space and time, as opposed to a particle that exist at only one point at a time.
Frequency	Number of complete cycles per second.
Galaxy	A group of billions of stars like our sun.
Ganesha	Names for the elephant-headed God, son of Lord Shiva.
Ganapati	Lord Ganesha.
Ganga	The holy river Ganges.
Gopi/ Gopis or Gopika	The milkmaids of *Brindavan,* companions and devotees of Sri *Krishna.*
Grahasthi	Married who lives with family. Householder.
Granthi	The psychic Knot in Braham Nadi, difficult to pierce by the Kundalini.
Gunas	Primary qualities of a human being: peaceful *(sathva),* active *(rajas)* and dull *(tamas).*
Guru	Spiritual teacher and a guide to spiritual path for a God seeker.
Hanuman	One of the most miraculous and devoted *bhakta* of Lord Rama represented as monkey man, mentioned in the *Ramayana.* He is still alive and gives His *Darshan* to His disciples.
Hatha yoga	School of yoga, which gives more importance to a*sanas* or yoga postures for the purpose of physical well-being and for awakening of the spiritual centers.
Hiranya-garbha	The cosmic source of life-energy.
Ida	A Nadi running to the left from the left side to Aggyia Chakra.
Indra	The king of the gods.
Involution	Involution means going back of the creation back to God. For every process of evolution (going away from God) there is a process of involution. The process of involution is going at

GLOSSARY

	all the time. At the end of the universe the whole creation will dissolve back in God. That will be a complete involution of the universe.
Jagat	The objective, transitory, untrue world.
Japa, japam	Recitation or repetition of the name of the Lord continuously.
Japamala	A religious necklace of 108 beads used *in japa* & repetition of the name of God with reverence and devotion.
Janam-asthmi	Festival in memory of the birth of Lord Krishna.
Kali	The ferocious black female diety.
Kama	Lust for sex.
Kanda	The source of all Nadis
Karma	Material activities with fruits of actions.
Karmic-law	The fruits of human actions are as per law of karma. The actions of God (lila) are without any fruits.
Karamphals	The fruits of actions.
Kirtan	Repetition of the name of lord with devotion in a group in the glory of God with classical music.
Knowledge	Opposite of *Maya* or ignorance, helps in knowing God and absolute truth.
Kriya Yoga	A scientific technique of special pranayam in seeking God promoted by Mahavtar Babaji.
Kumbhak	Inhalation of breath.
Kundalini	It is the individual creative Cosmic Energy of human known as serpent power. It is the female counter part of manifested God. When awakened it is responsible for the self-realization.
Kurukshetra	The battlefield of Mahabharata.
Lobh	Greed
Jal	Spiritually pure water like Ganga-Jal.
Ji	A syllable added to a word to denote respect,

	e.g., *Swamiji, Babaji*.
Jivan-mukthi or Moksha or Nirvana	The God-realized person in whom only the divine vision is active. He no longer has any identification whatsoever with his body. He is one with God.
Jnana or Gyana	Knowledge. The *yoga* path in which emphasis is laid on knowledge and discrimination, leading to wisdom, and the awareness of one's identity with the divine.
Jnani	One who has direct knowledge of the highest wisdom. One who follows the path of yoga. The word is also used to denote: one who has reached awareness of his divine identity.
Jyoti	The light and form of a flame.
Kailash	A peak of the Himalayas regarded as the sacred abode of Lord *Shiva*.
Kali or Mahakali	A name of the divine goddess mother; the Primal energy.
Karamphals	Accumulated fruits of past actions
Karma & Karmic-Law	Action; the law that governs all action and its inevitable consequences on the doer; the law of cause and effect, or moral compensation for acts done in the past.
Kirtan	Singing of spiritual songs by a group of devotees in the glory of God.
Kosas	The five sheaths of embodiment.
Krishna	An *Avatar (incarnation)* of *Vishnu*. Born nearly 5320 years ago in the end of Dwapara yuga.
Kumbhak	Retention of breath
Kundalini	Spiritual energy lying dormant in individuals at the lowest point of the spinal cord. It is different from *prana*. Without awakening Kundalini, there cannot be any process of involution (journey back to God)
Law of Cause & Effect	Every effect or an event must have a cause. There cannot be any event without any

GLOSSARY

	cause.
Laya Yoga	The techniques of concentration on *Anahat* sounds to achieve self-realization.
Leela (lila)	Divine play of God or His actions, which are without the fruits of karmas. The word is used to mean divine miracles also. But the whole of creation, being regarded as an inexplicable miracle, sometimes called the Lord's *lila*.
Life Energy or prana	Prana, Intelligent cosmic energy responsible for creation and organization of life and matter.
Light Year	Distance traveled by light in one year.
Lokas	As per scriptures there are 14 Lokas. Their names are Satya-Loka, Tapo, Janar, Mahar, Rudra, Vishnu, Bhu, Atala, Sutala, Nitala, Gambistha, Mahatal, Sutal and Patal.
Maha-Samadhi	Willfully leaving the body by the soul of a Yogi (willful death).
Mahatma	A great purified soul.
Mahavtar Babaji	The great grand guru of Sri Paramhansa Yogananda. The Eternal Himalayan Yogi.
Magic	A mysterious performance by using hidden tricks to deceive the viewers.
Maharishi Aurobindo	1872-1950: His ashram at Pondicherri, in Southern India, was turned into a community of spiritual seekers from all over the world, called Auraville. A prolific writer, his works include *The Life Divine, Essays on the Gita, The Synthesis of* Yoga, *Letters* on Yoga, and many others.
Mahima	The praise of superhuman power.
Manas	The mind.
Manav	Man. Human.
Mandir	Temple. A monument for the worship of God.
Manipur	A Chakra near the novel centre in the spine.

Chakra	
Mantra	Sacred words or verse repeated during meditation or Vedic hymn. Mantras are the power of the divine in the form of sound, word and letters. It is that which is the culture of true knowledge for getting rid of worldly fetters.
Margi	Path, road, way, course.
Mass	The quantity of matter in a body; its inertia; or resistance to acceleration.
Mauna	Observing silence.
Maya	Cosmic Delusion, Ignorance obscuring the vision of God; the primal enticing illusion appearing as duality and called the world; creates attachment with world.
Medulla Oblongata	The top end of the spine in the centre of skull. Seat of Soul, "Mouth of God".
Mind	The cosmic energy by which the brain functions
Miracle	A mysterious phenomenon generally seems to defy the known laws of sciences.
Moha	Attachments
Mukti or Moksha or Nirvana	Salvation or Liberation of soul free from material existence of birth and rebirth.
Mula	Origin, root, base.
Muladhar Chakra	A Chakra at the lower end of the spine. Seat of Kundalini.
Nad or Nada	Sound
Nadis	The nerves in the astral body that carries prana. Main Nadis are Ida, Pingla & Sushumana.
Nagar-Sankirtan	Nagar means city. Sankirtan means singing *bhajans or songs along with dance in the glory of God,* in a group while walking slowly through the streets; done in the early hours before dawn.
Narada	The ancient *rishi* or seer who wrote the classic

GLOSSARY

	of *bhakti yoga,* called *Narada Bhakti Sutras.*
Nauli	Purificatory exercise for abdominal region.
Neti	The exercise of cleaning of nostrils.
Neutrino	An extremely light elementary particle of negligible mass.
Neutron	Neutral particles like protons in the nucleus of an atom.
Neutron star	A cold star of mass little more then sun, which have a radius of few kilometers with a density of hundreds of millions of tons per cubic inch.
Niyama	Religious Observances.
Nirvikalpa Samadhi	When experiences total oneness with God & Truth after the death of ego 'I'.
Nirgun & Sugun	Nirgun means devoid of any properties (Brahman). Sugun means which have some properties. Nirgun is opposite of Sugun.
Nirvana or Moksha	Freedom from material existence. But still may be separate from God.
Nostradamus	A French doctor, who predicted thousands of major world events. He dreamed the future of the world.
Om or Aum	The primeval *Anahat* sound by which God sustains the cosmos.
Padma	Lotus. A name for plexus.
Padmasana	A cross-legged posture for long meditation.
Paramatma	The pure *atma* viewed in its universal aspect as God.
Paramhansa	The highest degree of spiritual achievement of Nirbhikalpa Samadhi. Higher then Swami.
Patanjali	The name of the ancient sage who wrote the basic guide to Y*oga,* known as *Patanjali Yoga Sutras.*
Photon	A quantum of light energy.
Pingla	Sun Nadi that runs on the right side of spine.
Positron	Positively charged antiparticle of electron.
Prakiriti	Primordial Nature, which in association with

	Purusha (eternal conscious principle) creates the universe.
Prana	The vital force or cosmic energy that sustains life in the physical body in all living beings. There are five types of *prana*.
Pranayama	Controlling the Prana with the regulation of breath.
Prasanthi Nilayam	The abode of undisturbed peace. The name of Sathya Sai Baba's *ashram* in India.
Prema	Divine love of the most intense kind, universal unconditional unblemished love. It is different from sexual lust generally called love.
Prema-rasa	The flavor (rasa) of *prema* (love).
Proton	Positively charged particle, which resides inside the nucleus of the atom.
Pundit	Scholar of the knowledge of God.
Puraka	Retaining the breath in lungs.
Puranas	Eighteen Holy Books of Hindu *Shastras*, which describes historical events and are supplements to Vedas. These are not mythology as said by some western Historians having no knowledge of Hindu *Shastras*.
Purusha	Eternal conscious principle; Soul.
Radha	The beloved & devotee of Lord *Krishna*.
Rajsic	The active, passionate aspect like king.
Rakshasas	The human race having *tamsic* characteristics.
Rama	An *Avatar* of God Vishnu in Treta-Yuga, a divine being. An *Avatar* whose name means, he who pleases; he who fills with *ananda* (bliss).
Ramakrishan Paramhansa	1836-1886: A great saint of Bengal. He was the spiritual guru of Swami Vivekananda.
Rechaka	Exhalation of breath.
Riddhi	Minor occult powers acquired by the yogis in the beginning. Yogis are able to perform minor miracles with these powers.

GLOSSARY

Rishi	A sage, one leading a life without desires, with attachments only to the a*tma*. A seer of truth.
Sabhikalpa Samadhi	The initial state of samadhi in which the yogi is aware of his ego 'I' separate from God.
Sacrum	Triangular shaped hollow bone situated below the pelvic region.
Sadhak	A spiritual aspirant engaged in conquering his egoism and greed, the sense of 'I' and 'mine'.
Sadhana	Spiritual discipline or practice through activities such as meditation and recitation of holy names.
Sadhu	A holy-man, generally used with reference to a monk.
Sahasrar	The thousand-patelled chakra in the forehead, which is the reservoir of life energy.
Sai	The divine mother of all.
Samadhi	An ecstatic state in deep meditation. It is the highest step on the eightfold path of Patanjali-Yoga. The shuttle experiences beyond delusion and Maya. Samadhi is attained when the meditator or observer, the process of meditation and the object of meditation (God) becomes the same. Trance, perfect equanimity, untouched by joy, sorrows and communion with God. Complete absorption in God consciousness.
Sankhya	One of the five attitudes cherished by the dualistic worshipper toward his chosen ideal: One of the six systems of Hindu philosophy.
Samsara or Sansara	The sensory world, which captures consciousness and gives rise to craving, attachment and suffering.
Samskaras	The tendencies inherent from previous births.
Sanathana Dharma	The ancient wisdom, the eternal path of righteousness.
Sankalpa	God's resolved or will.
Sankirtan	Reciting or singing devotional songs with joy.
Sanyasi or	A Hindu ascetic; one who has adopted the

Sanyias	monastic, celibate life. Wears saffron clothes. Do not live in any family.
Satan	*Maya.* The power by which God has separated Him from His creation.
Sathya Sai Baba	The most miraculous Avatara saint at Puttaparthy in India.
Shastras	The scripture that illumines, the moral code, directly transferred to humanity from God. Ordinary human mind cannot write *Shastras*, without the grace of God. Only superhuman man writes the Shastras. Shastras are the authority in the spiritual field.
Sat-chit-Ananda	The supreme state, usually translated as existence, knowledge, bliss.
Shat-karmas	Six purificatory exercises of Hath Yoga viz. Dhauti, Basti, Neti, Nauli, Trataka, and Kapalbhati.
Satwik	Pure, good, pious; the principle of balance or wisdom.
Sathya	Truth that which is always the same no matter past, present, future or circumstance
Satsanga	Being in the society of good, spiritual people.
Satwik, Rajas, Tamas	The three *gunas* or characteristics of embodied beings, translated roughly as peaceful, active and dull.
Savak	Devotee dedicated to the service of God.
Self	*Atman* or soul.
Self-Realization	The state of knowing God, the absolute state achieved by God, the soul merges in God and all the powers of God like omnipresent, omnipotent and omniscient are achieved Yogis when the body, mind and soul become one with The soul is in permanent Bliss or Happiness or Joy.
Shankar-acharaya	India's most advance self-realized saint. A great scholar, thinker and spiritual philosopher. He

GLOSSARY 247

	founded the four *Maths* (monastic centers of spiritual education) in India. The Head of the Math is known as *Jagadguru* (world teacher) Shankaracharaya.
Shakti or Adi-Shakti	The creative divine power; a name of the divine mother; the feminine aspect of God, representing His power and energy.
Shanti	Undisturbed peace, eternal peace.
Satwik	Pure.
Shirdi-Sai Baba	Great Indian holy man, worshiped both by Hindus and Muslims, from whom Sathya Sai Baba of Puttaparthy says he was reincarnated.
Shiva	Adi-Purusha. The destroyer God of the Hindu trinity, the other two being *Brahma* and *Vishnu*.
Siddha/ Sidhpurusha	A *siddha* is one who has attained *siddhies* (yogic *powers)*. Individualized Spirit. Perfect yogi.
Siddhi	Siddhis are the advanced powers of riddhis. These are eight in numbers: *Anima, Mahima, Laghima, Garima, Prapti, Parkamya, Vasitvam and Ishatvam.*
Spiritual eye	The third eye of Shiva or the single eye of intuition and omnipresent perception at the Aggyia chakra or between the eyebrows. When a yogi is under deep meditation the spiritual eye is visible. This is not present in the physical body.
Soham	So means He, and ham means I. Soham means He is I or I am He. This mantra is realized in Nirvikalpa samadhi.
Soul	Atma
Sri Raman Maharishi	1879-1950: He was an illumined *rishi* of southern India; taught non-duality through self-inquiry one should constantly ask oneself, "Who am I". His *ashram* is located on a sacred

	hill called *Arunachala*.
Sub-atomic particles	The elementary particles smaller then atom. There are more then 100 such elementary particles in the universe
Sukhasana	A cross-legged easy posture for meditation.
Swami	Lord, spiritual preceptor, a member of India's most ancient monastic order
Sutra	Aphorism.
Swadhisthan Chakra	The chakra near the Lumber in spine.
Swarupa/ Swaroopa	Form, body.
Tamas	Inertia, darkness.
Tamsik	Dull, lazy.
Tapa or Tapasya	Religious austerity, sacrifice, asceticism designed to weaken the conviction that man is body.
Tatvamasi	'Tatvam' means You (God) and asi means 'I'. This mantra means You and I are one. No duality.
Tratak	Gazing at a particular point. Concentration.
Treta Dwapara & Kali Yugas	The second of the four *yugas* or cycles of world periods. Hindu Shastras divides the duration of the world into four *yugas*, *Satya*, *Treta*, D*wapara* and Kali. The first is known as the Golden Age as there is a great preponderance of virtue among men, but with each succeeding *yuga* virtue diminishes and vice increases. In the Kali yuga there is a minimum of virtue and a great excess of vice. We are supposedly in the Kali *yuga* now. It was started after Lord Krishna approx. 5300 years ago.
Trikala Darsi	A person who knows the past, present and future.
Upadesh	Spiritual instruction.

GLOSSARY

Upanishad	A category of Indian scriptures. 108 philosophical treatises that appear within the *Vedas*.
Vedanta	Anta means end of Vedas or later portion of Vedas"; Adi Shankaracharaya was the chief exponent of Vedanta.
Vishuddha	Laryngeal plexus at the base of the throat.
Vritti	Mental function.
Yoga	Yoga means communion of *atma* (soul) with God. Yoga is that science by which the soul gains mastery over the instruments of body and mind and uses them to attain Self-realization— the reawakened consciousness of its transcendent, immortal nature, one with Spirit.
Veda	The Knowledge of God. The oldest scriptures about God are known as Veda.
Vedanta	One of the six systems of Hindu philosophy, formulated by Bhagwan Ved-Vyas.
Vedas	The most sacred scriptures of the Hindu religion, regarded as revelations to great seers and not of human origin. There are four main *Vedas:* The *Rig-Veda,* the *Yajur-Veda,* the *Sam-Veda* and the *Athar-Veda.* There are many more Vedas: Ayur-Veda, Dhanur-Veda, Gandharva-Veda and Sthapatya-Veda.
Vedic	Which is derived from Vedas.
Vibhuti	Sacred ash, frequently materialized by Sri Sathya Sai Baba.
Vishnu	The preserver God of the Hindu Trinity, the other two being *Brahma* and *Shiva.*
Vishuddha Chakra	The chakra in the spine near the cervical.
Yama	Moral conduct.
Yoga or Yog	Union of the individual soul with God; also the technique by which to realize this union. It is

	the general term for the several types of devotional practice that the disciplines used to control the mind and transforms it into an instrument for God-realization.
Yogi	The devotional spiritual aspirant who seeks union with God by means of one or more specific mental and physical disciplines which are traditional and which are known by the title of *yoga*.
Yugas	These are the four phases of world through which life moves to complete a world cycle. As per the scriptures their names and length of period in human years are: Sat-Yuga (17,28,000), Treta Yuga (12,96,000), Dwapara-Yuga (8,64,000) and Kali-Yuga (4,32,000). In Kali-Yuga we have passed nearly 5132 years.

Bibliography

The Name of Book	Author	Publisher
The Autobiography of a Yogi	Sri Paramhansa Yogananda	Jaico Publications, India.
The Men's Eternal Quest	-Do-	Yogoda Satsang Society of India, Ranchi & Self-Realzation Fellowship, USA.
The Divine Romance	-Do-	-Do-
Geeta Vahini	Sri Sathya Sai Baba	-Do-
Jnana Vahini	-Do-	-Do-
Dhyana Vahini	-Do-	-Do-
Pathways to God	Jonathan Roof	-Do-
Bhagwad Geeta	Bhagwan Ved-Vyas	Geeta-Press Gorakhpur, U.P. India
Manu-Smarity	Maharishi Patanjali	-Do-
Kaliyan Bhavishiya Puran	Ved-Vyas Compiled	-Do-
How to be Self-Reliant	Swami Ram Sukh Das	-Do-
Prana	Swami Vivekananda	Sri Ram-Krishan Mission, India.
The Awakening of Kundalini	Gopi Krishna	Kundalini Research Foundation, New York
The Evolutionary Energy in Man	Gopi Krishan	Shambhala Publications, Boulder, Colorado
Third Eye and Kundalini	Dr. B.S. Goel Siddheswar Baba	The Third Eye Foundation of India, New Delhi

Title	Author	Publisher
Holy Bible	New King James Version	India Bible Literature Beracah Road, Madras.
Way to Self-Realization	Sh.N.C. Kancil	Edu. Publisher Model Basti, New Delhi-5.
Chit-Shakti Vilas	Swami Muktananda	Gurudev Siddhapeeth Maharashra, India.
Bhagavad-Gita As It Is.	Swami Prabhupada	The Bhaktivedanta Book Trust
Journey to Self-Discovery	-Do-	-Do-
The Benefits of Fasting	Sh. Vithal Das Modi	Arogiya Mandir Prakashan
Dhyana Path	Sri Sidheshwar Baba	Third Eye Mission Bhaigan, Sonepat
Kundalini Yoga	Swami Shivananda	The Divine Life Society Shivananada Nagar, UP.
Tantra Yoga, Nada Yoga, Kriya Yoga	-Do-	-Do-
Hidden Mysteries of Kundalini	R. Venu Gopalan	B. Jain Publishers Paharganj, New Delhi.
Kundalini for Beginners	Dr. Ravindra Kumar	-Do-
Divine Shakti Kundalini	Swami Vishnu Tirtha	Yogshree Peeth Trust Rishikesh, India.
Kundalini and Meditation	Arjan Das Malik	Manohar Publishers & Distributors
History of the Tantric Religion	N.N. Bhattacharyya	-Do-
Healing with Form Energy and Light	Tenzin W. Rinpoche	New Age Books
Kundalini Tantra	Satyanada Saraswati	Bihar School of Yoga Munger, Bihar
Memories Dreams Reflections	Jung C.G.	Random House

Bibliography

Further Prophecies of Nostradamus	Cheetham Erika	Bantam Books New York
Soundarya Lahiri	Adi Shankar-acharya	--

About Saints & Authors

Sri Amar Jyoti Babaji	An incarnation of Maha Avatar Babaji, Mahavtar Babaji Ashram, Palampur, Himachal Pradesh, India.
Dr. B.S. Goel	Known as Siddeshwar Baba, Founder of Third Eye Foundation of India. Author: 'Third Eye and Kundalini'. Disciple of Sri Satya Sai Baba.
Swami Satyananda Saraswati	Author: 'Kundalini Tantra'. Founder: Bihar School of Yoga Munger, India.
Swami Shivananda	Author: 'Kundalini Yoga'. Founder: Divine Life Society, Shivananda Nagar, Rishi Kesh, Haridwar.
Swami Muktananda	Founder: Gurudev Siddhapeeth Maharashra India.
Gopi Krishna	Author: 'The Awakening of Kundalini' & 'The Evolutionary Energy in Man'.
Sri Paramhansa Yogananda	Founder: SRF California & YSS India. Author of: 'The Autobiography of a Yogi', 'The Men's Eternal Quest', and 'The Divine Romance' and many other spiritual books.

INDEX

Term	Pages
Aggyia Chakra	65, 88, 90-1, 188-90, 233, *
Aham-Brahmasmi	83, 233, *
Ahankar	233, *
Akasha or Ether	233, 237, *
Anahat Chakra	53, 88, 90-2, 185-6, 233, *
Anahat Sounds	53, 92, 233, *
Ananda	233, *
Ardha-Matsyendra	108
Asana	15, 99-110, *
Astral body	234, *
Astral-world	234, *
Atma/ Soul	234, *
Aum (Om)	100, 151, 231-2, 241, *
Aurobindo	241
Avatar / Avatara	234
Bandhas	112-117, *
Basti	122-3
Bhagavad-Gita	235, *
Bhakta / bhakti	73-76, 235, *
Bhastrika Pranayama	130
Bhujang Asana	108
Brahma	199, 231-2, 245, *
Brahma Granthi	199-200
Brahmachari	236, *
Brahmacharya	236, *
Brahman	231-2, 236, *
Brain	41
Causal body	236, *
Chakra	87-96, 167, 180-1, 236, *
Concentration	145-52, *
Death	86, *
Delusion	236, *
Desires	236, *
Devotion & Love	50, 73-76, 153, *
Dhanur-Asana	108
Dharana	17, 236
Dharma	236, *
Dhauti	122
Dhyana/ Meditation	237, *
Diksha	237, *
Dissolution in God	230
Dr. B.S. Goel	165, 173-4
Dr. Ravinder Kr	173-4
Dream	*
Dus-Karmas	237, *
Dwapara Yuga	237, *
Ego 'I'	23, 58, 66-72, 83 *
Ether	237, *
Evolution from God	228
Exercises	111-112
GRF	228
Ganesha	238
Gayatri Mantra	224
Gopi Krishan	173

* - Frequently repeated

INDEX

Grahasthi	238, *	Kundalini	20-24, 32-38, 141-3, 240, *
Granthi	46, 197-205 246, *	Law of Cause & Effect	240, *
Gross Body	230		
Gross Elements	230, *	Laya Yoga	53, 151-2, 241, *
Gunas	238, *	Leela or Lila	241, *
Guru	140, 220, 238,*	Life Energy or Prana	41-2, 77-96, 241, *
Hal-Asana	103		
Hanuman	175-6, 238, *	Lobha or Lobh	239, *
Hatha yoga	238, *	Lokas	241
Hiranyagarbha	238	Magic	241, *
Ida Nadi	80-83, 90, 238, *	Maha-bandha	114
Involution	20-23, 141, 228, *	Maha-Mrituanjia Mantra	220
Jal Neti/ Neti	136-7	Maha-Mudra	114
Jalandhara Bandha	133-4	Maha-Samadhi	241, *
Japa, Japam	239, *	Mahavtar Babaji	63-66, 154-8, 243, *
Jivan-Mukti	240, *	Manipur Chakra	88-90, 93,183-5,*
Jung C.G.	25, 34, 58	Mantra for Planets	221-3
Kali or Mahakali	220-21, 239		
Kali-Yuga See Dwapara	237	Mantra of Laxmi	220
		Mantras	215-226, 241, *
Kama	239, *	Matsya-Asana	102
Kapalbhati	127	Mauna	242, *
Karamphals	240, *	Maya	20-26, 242, *
Karma	240, *	Meditation	16-28,144-58, *
Khechari Mudra	116	Medulla Oblongata	79, 87-9, 242, *
Kirtan	240 *		
Krishna	240, *	Merudand Asana	110-1
Kriya Yoga	61-76, 150-8, 239, *	Mind	20-24, 41,122, *
		Miracle	242, *
Kumbhak	239, *		

* - Frequently repeated

INDEX

Misconceptions of Awaken Kundalini	170-174, *	Pratyahara	16, *
Moha	242, *	Psychologists	25
Moksha/ Mukti	244, *	Puraka	244, *
Mudras	112-117, *	Puranas	244, *
Mukti or Moksha	242, *	Rajas/ Rajsic	42, 244, *
Mula Bandha	112	Rakshasas	244, *
Muladhar Chakra	40, 88-90, 94, 180-1, 242, *	Rama	244
Nadi Suddhi	129	Ramakrishan Paramhansa	244
Nadis	80-3, 89-90, 135, 242, *	Dr. Ravinder Kr	182
Nauli	124	Rechaka	244, *
Nirgun/ Sugun	238, *	Reiki	133-6
Nirvana	253, *	Renunciation	26-28, *
Nirvikalpa Samadhi	18-20, 191-2, 243, *	Riddhi	176-9, 244, *
Niyama	12-4, 66-7, 212-3, 243, *	Rishi	244, *
Nostradamus	243	Rudra Granthi	201
Om or Aum	73-4, 133-4, 151-3, 232, *	Sabhikalpa Samadhi	18-20, 245, *
Padmasana	101-2, 243, *	Sahasrar	88-90, 190-1, 245, *
Paschimottan-Asana	105	Samadhi	18-20, 245, *
Patanjali	13-19, 150-3, 243, *	Samskaras	245, *
Piercing Kundalini	180-191, *	Sankirtan	245
Pingla Nadi	80-3, 90, 243, *	Sanyasi/ Sanyias	245, *
Plavini	145	Sarvang Asana	102-3
Pranayama	36, 100-104, 126, 141-8, *	Sat-Chit-Ananda	246, *
Pranic Healing/ Reiki	133-6	Satyananda Srwt	36, 90, 173-4
		Sathya Sai Baba	246, *
		Satsanga	246, *
		Satwa / Satwik	49, 246, *

* - Frequently repeated

INDEX

Self-Realization	246, *	Tatvamasi	248, *
Shakti	39, 46, 49, 246, *	Tratak/ Concentration	248, *
Shakti Chalana	117		
Shaktipat	206-214, *	Treta, Dwapara & Kali Yuga	248, *
Shankaracharya	246, *	Trikala Darsi	248, *
Shastras/ Scriptures	246, *	Uddiyana Bandha	113
Shav-Asana	112	Ujjayi Pranayama	131
Shiva	198-201, 219-20 247, *	Upanishad	248, *
Sukha Purvaka	129	Vajra Asana	108
Sidheswar Baba Dr. B.S. Goel	165, 174	Vedanta	249*
		Vedas	249, *
Siddhi	175-179, 247, *	Vegetarian Food	49, *
Soham	247, *	Vishnu	219, 250, *
Spinal Column	79-80	Vishnu Granthi	200-1
Spiritual/Third Eye	247, *	Vishuddha Chakra	88-90, 92, 186-7, *
Sri Yantra	225-6	Yama	12, 249, *
Sub-Pranas	85-6, 89, 229, 243, *	Yoga	249, *
Sugun/ Nirgun	243, *	Yogi/ Aspirant	250, *
Sukhasana	101-2, 248*	Yog-Sutras	12-18, *
Suryabhedi Pranayama	132	Yugas	250
Sushumana	66-73, 79-3, 90-95, *		
Swadhisthan Chakra	72, 88-90, 94, 91 182-3,248, *		
Satyananda Saraswati	53, 182-3, 198		
Symptoms of Awaking	174-179		
Tamas or Tamsik	41, 49, 248, *		

* - Frequently repeated